Overcoming Binge Eating 2-in-1 Value Collection: Mindful + Intuitive Eating

Set Yourself Free From Overeating, Emotional Eating Disorder, Unhealthy Habits & Weight Loss Diets without Giving Up Any Food

Written by Nathalie Seaton

Table of Contents

YOUR FREE GIFTS

As a way of saying thanks for your purchase and to help you along your journey towards developing healthier eating habits, we've created free bonus resources that will help you get the best possible results:

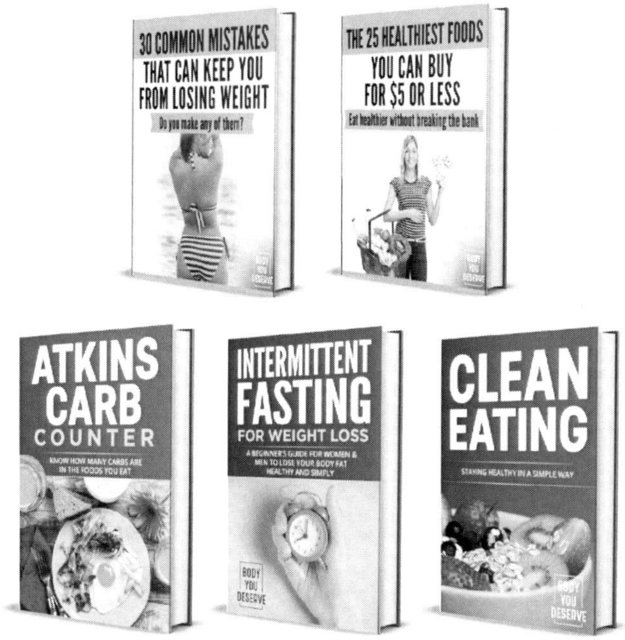

Free bonus #1: 30 Common mistakes that can keep you from losing weight
Do you make any of them?

Free bonus #2: The 25 Healthiest Foods You Can Buy for $5 or Less
Eat healthier without breaking the bank

Free bonus #3: Atkins carb counter
Know how many carbs are in the foods you eat

Free bonus #4: Intermittent Fasting for Weight Loss
A beginners guide for women & men to lose your body fat healthy and simply

Free bonus #5: Clean Eating
Staying healthy in a simple way

To get your bonuses, go to: http://bit.ly/NathalieSeaton

or scan with your camera:

Mindful Eating

Develop a Better Relationship with Food through Mindfulness,
Overcome Eating Disorders (Overeating, Food Addiction, Emotional and Binge Eating),
Enjoy Healthy Weight Loss without Diets

By Nathalie Seaton

Introduction

People come in all shapes and sizes and have their own history with food. They might be underweight, overweight, short, or tall. The media is flooded with advice on eating for specific body shapes, the best exercises, and the latest diet, but many people still have food battles. Regardless, the one constant for every person is that they have to eat, but the bigger question is why a person eats the way they do.

Eating habits are rooted in lifestyle and personality. The best way to consider eating habits is to think about the way you eat. Here are a few stories from other people regarding their eating patterns:

"I have always been a busy person running my own business, looking after the children, and taking part in several sports. I grab some quick snacks like carrot sticks or protein bars to keep me going, but I know I don't eat enough. When I do get time to myself, I will eat anything that is available, doesn't matter if it is bad or good. Afterward, I feel bad." - Amber, 42

"As children, my mother would dish up our food and we would eat every meal at the table. My parents were very strict, and we had to eat everything on our plates before we could get up from the table. I remember feeling full before I could finish my plate but I didn't have a choice of when to stop eating. This stretched my appetite, and I continued to eat larger portions as an adult. Now, I am overweight and wish I could change my situation." - Peter, 33

"I eat whenever I become stressed or emotional. I have been on too many diets to count and stick to them quite well, except when something bad happens. Then everything goes out the window, and I go back to my bad habits." - Mary, 27

Do you recognize yourself in the thoughts shared by Amber, Peter, and Mary?

So many people are trying to lose weight, gain weight, or improve their eating habits. It isn't easy, but change is possible. There is a way to consume food in a healthy way, without any feelings of guilt or shame, and enjoy it too! This method is mindful eating.

Mindfulness increases your awareness of the moment you are in and improves your appreciation of a current state. Mindful eating is an extension of this concept. It allows you to immerse yourself in eating so that you can nourish your body and your soul. Mindful eating creates an appreciation for food, how it is grown and produced, and the eating process. During this time, you become more aware of your role in the context of food.

Mindful eating is not a diet plan—it is a lifestyle. With mindful eating, you become aware of the food experience through active participation. It allows you to view yourself in a different light while improving your relationship with food. Mindful eating is about appreciating every food moment, the benefit it brings to your body, and how it makes you feel. Becoming a mindful eater enables you to reduce food anxiety, deal with your emotions, and gives you the control rather than having food control you. It is suitable for the whole family because it isn't a diet that eliminates foods or restricts calorie intake.

Once you learn how to eat mindfully, you realize there are no right or wrong foods and you can enjoy all food to varying degrees. You learn to accept that you are unique, so your eating experience will be distinctive too. As a mindful eater, you have a choice of what to eat, and the control to focus on only the eating process to enhance awareness. By gaining this awareness, you become responsible for your own food choices and accept that you are the only one that can control your health and life. This empowers you to continue eating mindfully without giving in to your emotions or external influences.

Throughout this book, we will look at the principles of mindful eating, practical application, how to make it a part of your life, and address problematic eating behaviors. Mindful eating isn't difficult, but it is normal to stray occasionally. To make mindful eating easier, we will consider how small changes can have a big effect, so don't push yourself to become a mindful eater overnight. Instead, take your time to master the concepts that are easiest for you before moving onto other mindful eating strategies. Most importantly, this book will teach you to love yourself by looking after your health in the best way possible!

Jan Chozen Bays, an American pediatrician, and educator on mindful eating and Zen practices shares this thought: *"Mindful eating replaces self-criticism with self-nurturing. It replaces shame with respect for your own inner wisdom."*

Chapter 1: The Science of Eating

Eating is an enjoyable activity for most people. It provides nourishment and comfort which may be why you constantly seek food. Few people eat recommended portion sizes, especially if it is a beloved food. It is a huge challenge to eat healthy if you really love a specific food. Why is this the case? Understanding why you eat the way you do is the first step to understanding yourself better and dealing with your eating problems.

Eating is necessary for survival and your brain is hardwired to seek food for sustenance. In previous centuries, people would hunt and look specifically for food with higher calories (like bananas rather than tomatoes) to ensure they could do their daily tasks, but these activities were more physical than they are today. Today, people still choose higher-calorie foods, but the contextual lifestyle has changed entirely. Often, the foods that are the cheapest and are most readily available are packed with fat, sugar, and carbohydrates.

Besides the innate drive to eat for survival, people also forge emotional attachments to food. For example, your family might eat cake every Friday, have three course-meals for birthdays, or celebrate being the winning team with a couple of alcoholic drinks. All of these events make you feel good, and you cannot imagine those events without these consumption patterns. Similarly, you might crave the chicken soup your mother makes when you don't feel well because this nostalgic meal made you feel better. This emotional link to food is something that many people struggle with, but biology does have a bit to do with this situation.

A Biological Loop

Your brain sends signals to inform you that it wants to eat. When this happens, the hypothalamus, a part of the brain, triggers neurotransmitters and hormones that encourage you to eat. So, eating is a biological process. However, eating is something you are taught to do from the time you are born. The act of chewing and swallowing starts when you are an infant, and it provides satisfaction because you are answering the call of the hypothalamus.

As you eat, your stomach expands, and receptors send signals to your brain to indicate you are nearing fullness. This connection between your mind and body is known as the mind-gut connection. The receptors also trigger the release of feel-good hormones which makes eating a pleasant activity. One of these hormones is dopamine that rewards you for eating by providing feelings of pleasure which is why many people eat to feel better. The truth, though, is that feel-good hormones can be triggered by other activities than eating, so food should not be the only coping mechanism you use.

Reasons To Eat

Food is all around us, which means there is temptation and all the more reason to eat. People are eating more because food is convenient, accessible, and scientifically-engineered to make the eating experience enjoyable. This barrage of food information provides a challenge. Are you physically hungry or is it your mind and body playing tricks on you?

In most cases, you can classify your hunger into one of three categories. The first is a physical need to eat. If you are truly hungry, then you would be willing to eat anything. To determine if you are physically hungry, ask yourself whether you are willing to eat a carrot or something similar that is really healthy, specifically if it is not something you would normally choose. The second reason for eating is a desire or want to consume food. Usually, this desire comes across as cravings for something sweet, savory, carb-loaded, or textural. It is an experiential desire and not a pang of physical hunger. The final reason is believing you should eat, such as thinking you must eat because it is lunchtime or since other people are eating.

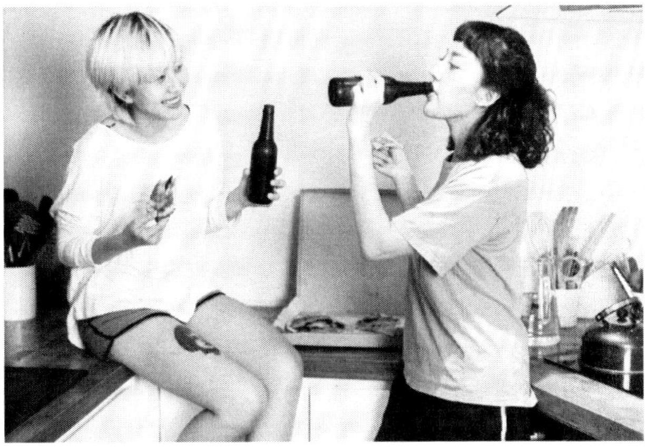

The Way We Eat

Now that you know the reasons why people eat, it is time to look at food prompts and the way we eat food. The media and grocery stores bombard shoppers with numerous food choices and include all kinds of scientific claims. Unfortunately, a lot of foods that are healthy are in stores either because it's expensive or people favor convenience foods. Let's see how all these factors come together to help us make food choices and get some insight into how mindful eating can help.

Taste Rather Than Health

Sometimes, people do not naturally choose food based on it being healthy. Rather, people prefer foods that taste good. For example, you might decide to eat an orange because it is sweet, not because it contains a lot of vitamin C. This desire for good taste is something you are born with and develops over time. Being exposed to a variety of foods as a child can make it easier for you to enjoy healthier foods, but in many cases, you will have to acquire a taste for healthy foods through the knowledge that it is good for you. Mindful eating will help you to increase your awareness of food and teach you to savor every bite.

Favorites

Everyone has a favorite food, and probably more than one. Your favorite food could provide a sense of nostalgia or conjure up good feelings, so you might eat this food more frequently. Many people struggle to give up their favorite foods when going on a diet and probably break their diet because they chose to eat a favorite. Having an obsession with these foods will prevent you from sticking to a diet, but mindful eating doesn't require that you give up any foods. Instead, you will learn how to enjoy your favorite foods in moderation while considering your health.

Diet Personality

You are a unique individual and have your own personality. You like certain foods prepared in specific ways, just like you have other eating habits. For example, you might eat three meals a day based on a meal plan or prefer six smaller meals per day. Changing your diet personality to fit in with a new diet is a challenge because you are used to doing things in a specific manner. Mindful eating does not require adaptations to your diet personality. It teaches you to use your diet personality mindfully, which is the key to weight management success.

Visual Consumption

The saying, "eating with your eyes" is one you may be familiar with. It means that looking at food already awakens your senses and makes you want to eat the food you see. Think about restaurant menus containing pictures, watching cooking shows, and food displays in the store. You naturally gravitate to the plates with visual appeal and find yourself salivating by simply looking at the dish. Food that looks good is a temptation, but mindful eating will help you decide whether you really need to eat that food or whether you can replicate a dish in a healthier way.

Choices Galore

Have you ever been to a buffet restaurant, or maybe had a buffet at a wedding? There are so many choices that you don't know what to pick, so you take a bit of everything. Think about the last buffet for a moment. If you took two types of meat, rice, roasted potatoes, three veg, salad, and two desserts, then you have eaten about three times the number of calories than you should in an average meal. This amounts to approximately the same number of calories as you would eat on an average day because buffets make you dish up larger portions too. In contrast, sticking with a few basic foods at mealtimes and avoiding buffets as far as possible is best. Mindful eating allows you to exercise control when choosing which foods to eat and enables you to eat less of the items on a buffet.

Convenience and Cost

People rush from one thing to the next, be it work, school, sports, or hobbies. This constant rushing and feeling tired limits your time and makes it difficult to think about and cook proper food. It is much easier to grab a coffee and bagel on the way to work, soda with a takeout meal, a sugary snack during your lunch break, and grab a frozen convenience meal on the way home. Sometimes, people feel that these options are faster and cheaper than making meals from scratch, but this is not always the case. With mindful eating, you will learn how to choose your food wisely so that it provides nutrition, but can also be put together quickly. If you become a mindful eater, you can make better decisions even when it comes to takeout and at restaurants, which makes it easier to eat healthily.

Boredom

Sometimes, people are bored and need something to do, so they reach for a snack. You probably have several examples of this in your own life which may include eating mindlessly while watching TV or snacking while lounging next to the pool. When you are bored, your mind seeks stimulation and a release of hormones, which is easy to achieve with eating. These activities and accompanied eating are not beneficial to your health or wellbeing. With mindful eating, you will realize that your boredom can be turned into productive activities that release feel-good hormones without a bite of food.

Social Eating

The average person eats substantially more when they are away from home, and especially when in the company of other people. Social gatherings tend to be loaded with food since several people bring dishes or snacks leading to more food than necessary for each person. Giving in and eating more than you should occur through an unsaid type of peer pressure when people offer food, or those around you over-consume, which lets your own guard slip. Mindful eating teaches you to savor the company instead of the food and encourages spending time with people that also make healthy choices.

A Scientific Dilemma

The media continuously reports about the latest diet trend, the best foods to eat, and ones you should avoid at all costs. A few months or years later, you read a new article in the same publication claiming that the food it once reported as the holy grail should now be avoided at all costs. Eggs are a great example of this phenomenon. During the 1990s and early 2000s, reports indicated that eggs are off-limits if you want to avoid heart problems. By 2015, dietary advice said that eggs are an excellent source of protein and can be eaten without cholesterol or cardiovascular worries. In 2019, the egg debate took another u-turn when studies showed a link between eggs and a higher chance of cardiovascular problems. There is so much conflicting information that it's hard to know what to do.

If science doesn't know what you should and shouldn't eat, then how should you know what is right and wrong? No wonder diet advice is contradictory—it really depends on who you ask for advice. There are a few reasons for this contradictory advice including our own food reporting, too many scientific variables and a good deal of marketing input.

Answering Questions

Questionnaires are a great source of information for researchers, but participants don't always answer truthfully. For example, if someone approaches you with a questionnaire about your caffeine habit, it is very difficult to admit that you drink six cups of coffee per day, so you rather select the option that says you drink two coffees daily. The next question could ask whether you consume energy drinks and how frequently. You don't want to admit you drink one energy drink daily because you think it will reflect badly on you.

The problem with answering questionnaires in this way is that you are distorting the research results. If the researchers surveyed 500 people and half of them changed their answers favorably, then that research is no longer useful, but the researchers don't know when someone isn't telling the truth. They analyze the data from this research and use it to provide dietary advice, but obviously, this advice has issues. No wonder some research claims seem ludicrous when reading articles. If you ever do participate in research, then ensure you answer truthfully because you will be helping other individuals just like yourself who look to researchers for dietary advice.

Too Many Variables

To test whether any food is great or problematic, researchers must do studies. A proper research study requires that the researchers control specific variables and compare them to a placebo or control group. It is very challenging to control all variables in a research study. For example, to study the effect of eggs on a person's health, researchers may require that participants eat no other proteins or fatty foods that could affect the heart. This is a huge challenge for participants, especially if they have to take control of their own meal plans.

The other issue is that each person is different, so studying the food effects in one group might not provide the same results in another group. For example, testing in a group of individuals with a body mass index (BMI) below 25 might not help individuals with a BMI over 30. Similarly, studying food effects in diabetics may not yield the same results as in individuals with no health problems. It is crucial that you understand the context of a research study before assuming it is applicable to your case.

Food Marketing

Every organization wants to push the sales of their products, so they turn to marketing to boost their numbers. Some food producers, including healthy food manufacturers, will pay researchers to do research into their products and cherry-pick results that provide favorable results. For example, a wine producer may pay for a study to show that their wine has health benefits but ignore the alcoholic effect. These results are published in the media and individuals seeking affirmation of their food choices will then purchase this product because it is deemed healthy. In reality, the results are distorted because they were purchased, just like manufacturers pay for advertising for other products. Always question the article if it contains words like “sponsored” or “paid promotion.”

Mindful Eating Encourages Healthy Eating

Every day, you are faced with a myriad of food choices, and there are many reasons why you might eat. This situation is entirely normal. Turning to research and dietary advice is useful, but may not provide the information you require. The great thing about mindful eating is that it doesn’t restrict food, rather, it encourages healthy eating habits. By focusing on your awareness while eating, you are addressing your emotions and concentrate on filling your body with good nutrients. It is a natural way to improve your life without worrying when a certain food will go out of fashion.

Chapter 2: Unhealthy Eating Behaviors

What eating habits do you have that you consider unhealthy? You might consider a bad eating habit to be skipping breakfast, adding extra butter to your toast, or sneaking midnight snacks. The main issue is that society is okay with encouraging a fast-casual trend, and you fall victim to this lifestyle since instant gratification seems easier than taking time to prepare and eat food.

Fast-casual dining may seem like a quick fix when you are running around to get everything done, but it creates three major issues. First, you cannot enjoy your food if you are eating quickly, which leaves you craving more since you remain unsatisfied. Secondly, consuming food and drinks mindlessly means you are on autopilot which tends to increase overeating. Finally, evolution changed your body to release digestive enzymes more slowly, but eating quickly does not allow your body to digest food properly. All of these issues create further health problems.

Signs of a Poor Diet

Most people think the first sign of a poor diet is a changing waistline or clothes that no longer fit properly, but there are many other signs that show up ahead of time. The following signs might be some you have experienced previously and could point to bad eating habits.

Straw-like Hair

When you eat, the nutrients from the food are distributed to your organs to let them function properly. Eating poorly means you get less of these essential nutrients. Hair follicles, where the hair root is situated in your head, are a type of organ too, so your hair gets insufficient nutrition. Starvation diets and eating foods with poor nutritional values decrease the protein available to your organs and hair which causes brittle hair, loss of pigmentations (gray hair), and hair loss. Your hair could feel dry, thin, or like straw if you do not consume proper nutrients.

Skin Problems

Dry, oily, or troublesome skin could be an indicator of poor health. Your skin requires sufficient nutrition to remain elastic and in good condition. Removing specific foods from your diet could result in dry skin, such as when you don't eat any healthy fats. Similarly, eating too much oily food may lead to skin breakouts and pimples. Any damage to your skin could cause premature aging and make your skin look dull, wrinkled, create dark undereye circles, or lose its glow. Eating a balanced diet allows your skin to receive the required nutrition to look great.

Digestive Changes

Digestive problems like reflux, constipation, and diarrhea are prevalent symptoms of a poor diet. Insufficient fiber is the usual culprit for both constipation and diarrhea and can affect your overall health. With mindful eating, you will learn how different foods contribute to your health and bodily functions. You will also realize that there are many food choices that provide excellent nutritional benefits, which means you rely less on chemically produced items to help ease your digestive problems.

Oral Health Issues

Cavities and gum problems are signs of a bad diet, especially if you practice good oral hygiene like brushing your teeth and flossing. Eating too many sugary foods or consuming fizzy drinks causes damage to the enamel of the teeth which may result in cavities. Your gums may have a red line where they meet the teeth or have inflammation or bleeding. These things indicate some type of gum infection, which is another indicator of bad health or nutritional deficiencies, such as too little vitamin C. Mindful eating improves your health by encouraging consumption of nutrient-rich foods while eating less junk food.

Poor Healing

Cuts or other wounds require protein, nutrients, and calories to heal properly and in good time. Eating poorly weakens your immune system, which means your wounds do not get what is necessary to heal quickly and well. Insufficient nutrition delays the generation of new tissues and creates an opportunity for infection. It is best to increase the consumption of nutritious foods to give your body a chance to heal properly.

Brain Drain

Any memory problems or feeling extremely tired could indicate a lack of adequate nutrition. If you do eat healthy foods, then your brain doesn’t receive the nutrients it requires to function. This causes fatigue, shortens your attention span, and makes you forget things. Mindful eating will teach you that eating healthily improves your mental health and makes it easier to sleep—it helps you to be mindful of everything you do, so you might find that you change your sleeping patterns too.

Getting Sick Frequently

Poor nutrition compromises our immune system leaving us susceptible to infection and illness. A weak immune system struggles to fight off infection, so it leaves you vulnerable to becoming ill easily, and you take longer to get better. Eating foods containing lots of vitamins and nutrients ensures your immune system gets a boost and strengthens your immune system to fight off future infections.

Bad Eating Habits

Sometimes, you remain unhappy with your body, even when you put in a conscious effort to improve yourself. You might want to put on a few extra pounds to become pregnant or lose a few pounds to fit into a special outfit. Regardless of the changes you make, you do not see the results you want. This can leave you feeling frustrated and unmotivated. The reason for this could be a bad eating habit and one you might not realize you have. The following list contains some of the most popular bad eating habits.

Mindless Eating

Mindless eating is something you might fall prey to. It occurs when you eat without concentrating on the food you are consuming, such as eating popcorn in a movie theater or snacking while working on a computer. You don't realize how much you are consuming when you do this, and you might be surprised that the bowl is empty when you can't even remember taking more than one or two bites. Another problem with mindless eating is the way you serve the food. Purchasing the largest size containers will result in eating more, especially if you eat straight from the packaging. Similarly, placing food in a large bowl or on a large plate makes it seem as if you have very little on your plate, so you will mindlessly eat everything and not appreciate the amount. Being mindful of food requires consideration of what you are eating and how you present it.

Skipping Breakfast

Breakfast gives you a start to your day and helps improve your concentration and energy. You might skip breakfast because you have too many other things to do. Skipping breakfast could lead to overeating later during the day or drinking energy drinks to get through the day. Mindful eating encourages you to do the best thing possible for your body, and that may include eating breakfast, which could help you to lose weight and have more energy in the long-term. However, you could find skipping breakfast beneficial if you are using the 16/8 intermittent fasting method, as it improves energy and concentration.

Nighttime Eating

Are you one of those people who wants a midnight snack, or opens the fridge frequently after dinner? Some research studies found that eating at night may cause weight gain. The other problem is that most nighttime snackers select starches or sugary foods that are high in carbohydrates. Your body needs less energy while you sleep, so all those consumed calories cannot be used productively, and you might experience poor sleep as your body digests the food. Mindful eating helps you to make better food choices and questions whether you are truly hungry, which means you might overcome this habit once and for all.

Insufficient Daytime Eating

Eating fewer meals during the day doesn't mean you will lose weight automatically. You might skip breakfast or lunch, because you are too busy to eat or think it will help you to lose weight, but the opposite tends to happen. If you skip meals, you may find you are snacking more, or become so famished that you consume too much food at night. You might even eat more than you would have on a typical day. Eating poorly throughout the day results in fluctuating energy levels, and may leave you feeling tired. Mindful eating helps you focus on the best nutrition for your body so that you are in your best shape possible.

Not Eating at Home

Buying foods from coffee shops, take-outs, or restaurants is a problem. Not only can it take bites out of your budget, but it also decreases your awareness of food. You might find that you order more than you would eat at home or choose foods high in fat and carbohydrates. Most places prepare huge portions which means you might be eating more than you should. Those extra calories quickly add up, especially if you frequent these establishments. The best option is to eat meals made at home and prepare your own food for work where you have full awareness and can make proper food decisions.

Frequent Snacking

Snacking is a big problem for many people. You might want something to munch between meals when you go from one appointment to the next or while driving. Although you might choose an apple or celery sticks occasionally, you most likely reach for a high-calorie item like cookies or donuts. Mindful eating will change this habit into questioning to decide if you really need to eat and the best thing to eat.

Emotional Eating

After a bad day, when you want to celebrate something, or during high-stress times, you may find yourself eating more. This is a coping mechanism to help you deal with your emotions. Sometimes, people call it "eating your feelings," which describes the situation quite well. Emotional eating frequently results in consuming more than you should or eating less nutritious foods. With mindful eating, you will finally get control over emotional eating and find other ways to cope with your feelings.

Quick Eating

You might have a hectic schedule and find it easiest to eat on the run by grabbing a sandwich between meetings or drinking an energy drink as a quick "pick me up" before heading to the gym. Few individuals who eat on the go make healthy food choices because the easiest option is to get convenience food or to grab a snack full of processed food items. Combined with eating on the go comes eating food rapidly. You only have a few minutes between meetings or while driving and need to eat your food in a short time. When you eat quickly, you don't give time for your stomach to communicate feelings of fullness to your brain, which means you eat much more before feeling full. Slowing down is a part of mindful eating that helps you to enjoy your food and become aware of satiation.

Improper Liquid Use

Drinking fluids is essential for hydration, but few people use liquids responsibly. It is best to drink water since it hydrates without adding extra calories. Think about what you drink on a daily basis. Many individuals drink sugary beverages, energy drinks, or excessive amounts of alcohol. All of these fluids contain extra calories, so mindlessly drinking liquids could become problematic if you are trying to be healthier. It is much better to select low-calorie beverages and enjoy the hydrating feeling rather than the instant gratification of other drinks.

Eating Alone

Life has become a constant rush, and many families no longer eat meals together. This is problematic because you might start eating at strange times of the day, eat too much, or skip several meals entirely. When you eat alone, you tend to take shortcuts or opt for convenience foods and snacks rather than eating healthy meals like you would have if you were eating with family. Make time to sit down with your family, or if you are far away from them, then have meals with your friends or neighbors. It encourages you to spend time together and improves your health, which means your eating habits improve too.

Portion Confusion

How do you decide what a suitable portion of food should be? Do you measure it out in weight or simply ladle the food onto your plate? Most people tend to misjudge portion sizes entirely and opt for larger sizes rather than a recommended daily amount. Restaurants and takeout establishments don't help this process either because they provide supersized portions. Although mindful eating doesn't limit your food choices, you should still consider whether the amount of food you consider as a portion is suitable, or whether it requires adjusting. In most cases, this will happen naturally during the mindful eating process through various techniques.

Junk Food

Plenty of processed foods can be found in takeaways shops and grocery store aisles. It includes any food that has gone through some form of processing, which usually has added ingredients. For example, chips, processed cheese, frozen chicken, candy, and so on. Processed food contains excess amounts of sugar, salt, and fat, and these are all bad for your health. You might not realize what is going into your food products if you don't read food labels. Junk food may contain ingredients that encourage addiction and trigger the release of feel-good hormones, which only makes you eat more.

Mindful eating improves awareness of ingredients in foods you select and encourages healthier options.

Sneaky Sugar

You may know there is sugar in candy, fizzy drinks, and cookies, but there is a lot of sugar in other foods too, even healthy ones. Salad dressings, bread, fruit juice, and whole-grain cereals along with many other foods, contain added sugar. Sugar adds large amounts of calories to your diet, but it holds no nutritional value, which means it is empty calories. Take some to be mindful about the foods you eat by reading the ingredients and food label to see if the food contains sugar. You might be surprised about how many foods have sugar and simply making better choices could have a great effect on your health.

Eating Continuously

You might find yourself eating continuously. For example, you grab some risks with your first coffee in the morning, have breakfast, eat lunch, grab something else to eat for extra energy at lunch, have dinner, and eat something small to last you for the last few hours of the night. Constant eating is different from snacking because you eat with the intention of having smaller meals to provide you energy, rather than eating something quickly. Most, if not all, of this frequent eating happens mindlessly. It makes food a crutch for support because you just need a little something to keep going.

Screen Time

Staring at a screen for hours on end can result in mindless eating and overeating. You might work a job where you are behind a computer screen for several hours a day, enjoy watching a series, spend time playing video games, or use your mobile phone frequently.

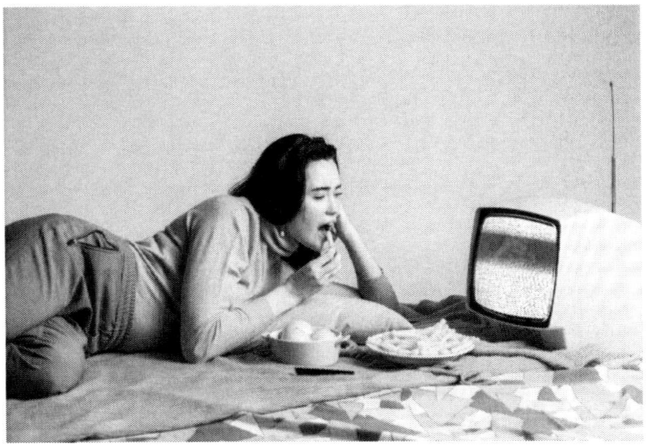

All of this screen time can be disastrous, especially if you are eating snacks in between, instead of preparing meals and eating with family members. If you have spent several hours in front of a screen, then you could be consuming much more when you do get your hands on food. Another issue is that you either drink too much or too little fluids, which causes excess calorie consumption in the first case and dehydration in the latter. Being mindful encourages an overall healthier lifestyle which means you will be eating better and moving more.

Not Planning Meals

The majority of people do not plan their meals. You might shop aimlessly and simply add more foods to the cart. Most of these foods are microwave or oven meals, junk food, or sugary snacks. Even worse, you might be so busy that you forgo making meals entirely, and rather opt for a drive-thru or meal delivery service. Many times, you might blame being busy for this situation. However, doing a meal plan only takes a few minutes and you can shop quickly because you know what foods you require. It will help you save time and money, and your body will thank you for feeding it less junk. Meal planning can seem like a chore, but it is an opportunity to become aware of what you are going to eat and whether it is good for you.

Healthy Food Trap

There are some misconceptions about so-called "healthy" foods. You might drink a protein shake and add some fruit and peanut butter into it, for example. Although all these foods are healthy, they contain lots of calories, fats, and sugars which quickly increases your calorie count for the day. This results in overeating and makes you feel uncomfortably full. Another example is eating a vegetable platter at a restaurant since vegetables are healthy. However, the added ingredients like oil, salt, and cream change the calorie count and you may not realize that the portions are too large, so you continue to overeat.

Poor Eating Affects Your Health

The signs of a poor diet already indicate that unhealthy eating already has consequences. However, those symptoms are minor when compared to some other potential consequences. Understanding the risks helps you to understand why eating healthy food is essential if you want to be the best possible version of yourself.

Obesity

Being overweight is a major concern for anyone with poor eating habits. All the junk you are feeding your body will add up, and eventually, it causes excess weight. This is something that almost two-thirds of Americans struggle with, which shows the extent of mindless eating. Obesity increases your risks of getting other medical conditions, so it is something you want to avoid.

Hypertension

Hypertension, commonly known as high blood pressure, is a big problem, since many people do not realize they suffer from this condition. You may experience hypertension if you eat a lot of junk food, sugar, salt, refined foods, and fried food. Even with treatment, hypertension may still result in cardiovascular issues such as heart attacks.

High Cholesterol

Foods that contain fat contribute to cholesterol levels in your body. Eating high-fat food, especially those with saturated fats, is the main culprit in this case, since it causes excess fat in your blood and affects your heart. High cholesterol levels could lead to blockages in your blood vessels and heart disease, which kills thousands of people each year.

Stroke

Plaque can build up in your blood vessels just like it does on your teeth. It is the result of eating foods high in cholesterol, fat, and salt. When this happens, your blood vessels become narrower and make it more difficult to pump blood through your body. When plaque build-up breaks free from a vessel, it forms a clot, which can travel through your circulatory system. Blood clots that enter the brain cause strokes, which could result in brain damage, impaired cognitive abilities, and death.

Diabetes

Although some cases of diabetes occur with a healthy diet, the majority of diabetes cases are caused by poor nutrition. Diabetes happens when you have too much sugar in your bloodstream or when your body cannot process sugar properly. Usually, eating large amounts of sugar and fat contribute greatly to diabetes, so simple dietary changes can help you address the situation. Diabetes frequently goes hand-in-hand with obesity which is another risk factor.

Insomnia

Insomnia refers to lying awake at night because you cannot sleep. Certain foods, such as those high in sugar and processed items, may cause insomnia, as they stimulate your brain activity and other bodily functions. If you do not sleep properly, then you may find yourself searching for a midnight snack, drinking more (meaning you have to get up and urinate frequently), or overeating at other times. Insomnia leaves you tired and causes concentration difficulties which affects your daily activities.

Gout

Gout is something that frequently appears after eating certain foods, such as red meat, specific seafood, and dairy products, among others. These foods could create a build-up of uric acid which forms crystals in joints like the knuckles and toes. As a result, the crystal causes inflammation and pain since they aren't supposed to be there in the first place. Continuous gout may lead to permanent joint damage—a big problem if you value your mobility.

Decreased Sports Performance

If you want to perform at your best, then you need to feed your body the best possible foods. Unfortunately, you might still choose junk food as a quick-fix before practice or after the gym. Junk food cannot provide the nutrients you need to keep up during sports resulting in decreased performance and fatigue. Additionally, poor nutrition decreases your healing rate after injuries, so your recovery will take longer, which takes you out of action for lengthy periods.

Are You Eating Mindlessly?

Throughout this chapter, you may have identified some of the symptoms and consequences of poor nutrition in yourself. If you are still uncertain about whether you eat mindlessly, then consider the following questions.

Do you:

- Frequently eat until you feel overly full or even to the point of becoming nauseous?
- Eat while doing other things (multitasking)?
- Graze on snacks without recognizing taste?
- Eat as quickly as possible?
- Struggle to remember how the food looked, tasted, or smelled soon after you finish eating?

If you answered "yes" to any of these questions, then you are guilty of some type of mindless eating. Luckily, this is not a permanent situation, as long as you are willing to change. Mindful eating is the perfect antidote for your consumption challenges.

Chapter 3: Mindful Eating Matters

What is the first thing you think of when you hear the words "mindful eating?" Some people think it requires meditation or giving thanks before taking a bite of food. You might associate mindful eating with taking a lot of time or having to sacrifice some foods. This is not the case at all. Mindful eating simply refers to concentrating on the food and your feelings while you eat. It increases your awareness while eating and enables you to understand your body's internal cues better.

Psychology and Mindful Eating

How you feel frequently affects all parts of consumption—what you eat, when you eat it, and why you eat what you do. Feeling good after eating is not a bad thing since you are nourishing your body, but it is the type of food you eat and the amounts that determine whether it is good or bad for you. Unfortunately, many people have unhealthy relationships with food, such as when you eat too much or too little, which means you associate food with negativity. Mindful eating encourages you to view food choices in a positive light by changing the way you make food-related decisions, regardless of your history with food.

Therapists believe that various elements in our past and present may affect our relationship with food. Culture, evolution, family, social settings, psychological issues, and economic status may influence your food choices. You might be part of a culture where every celebration is accompanied by food in excess and it is frowned upon to only eat small portions. In contrast, your friends may all be slim and peer pressure could force you to eat less food. You might also dislike certain foods if you grew up eating mostly that food due to financial constraints or your taste may be more expensive, because you come from a wealthy family. Each person and their eating habits are unique, so don't force yourself to fit the mold.

Psychology considers how you behave including your behavior towards food. All the factors above may cause specific behaviors and therapists frequently help people to overcome food problems by addressing these actions. Weight management requires behavioral and cognitive interventions if you want to succeed in reaching your goal. Behavioral treatment is used to identify your eating patterns and to determine methods that will alter this pattern. Cognitive treatment refers to thinking with the aim of identifying destructive thinking patterns that may contribute to body dysmorphia or weight problems. Most therapists use strategies that combine behavioral and cognitive concepts to help you overcome your weight challenges.

Readiness For Change

Before you can change, you have to be willing to change. Usually, psychologists will work on getting you ready for change first, so that you can understand what you need to do to reach your goals. This may include writing a list of weight objectives and making a conscious decision to commit to this change.

Self-Monitoring Acuity

Monitoring your food choices and weight management progress is essential and can help you stay motivated. Writing down what you are consuming or how you feel will make you more aware of your decisions and help you to identify trends or behaviors. Monitoring your progress provides you with a comparison tool to help you see how far along you have come.

Breaking Stimulus Control

Therapy helps you to break the hold that food, emotions, and events have over your eating habits. This could be something as simple as removing bad food choices from your home or staying away from dining out. Distraction is another therapy that helps to release you from the bonds of food by replacing it with other options such as reading a book or going for a walk. Positive reinforcements, like affirmations, finding a friend to support you, or rehearsing troublesome food scenarios may assist in sticking to your weight management plan too.

From Negative to Positive

A large part of behavioral cognitive techniques focuses on being positive rather than negative. Your thoughts are a powerful tool that you can use for good or bad, so concentrating on positive thoughts during weight management is essential. For example, your default thought might be, "I don't like the way my body looks," but this can change to a positive thought such as, "I am working towards a better version of myself."

Science and Mindful Eating

Mindful eating is based on science, as seen in the first chapter with the biological influence between mind and stomach. Science has also proven that mindful eating is useful for weight management, so it could work for you too. In 2017, the Nutrition Research Reviews journal published several articles about mindful eating. The review indicated that mindful eating tends to "rewire" the brain to break bad eating habits and replace them with good habits. When attached to neurofeedback devices, the researchers found that mindful eaters had less activity in the part of the brain that controls cravings and emotional eating.

Having fewer cravings means you could lose weight through mindful eating. *The Journal of Family Medicine and Community Health* reported that a 15-week mindful eating weight loss study during 2018 resulted in behavioral changes and weight loss for participants. Participants that used mindful eating practices dropped six times as much weight when compared to a control group. The researchers also found that participants from the mindful eating group continued to use these techniques when questioned six months after the study. This shows that increasing awareness can go a long way to changing behaviors.

The journal, *Obesity*, published a 2016 article about a mindful eating study. One group of participants received coaching regarding mindfulness, proper diet, and exercise plans, while the other group got no mindfulness training. The aim of this study was to understand the impact of mindful eating on a person's health, rather than on only weight loss. During the study, mindful-eating participants ate fewer sweets and continued with this behavior when questioned on a follow-up appointment. Reducing their sugar intake resulted in lower cholesterol and fasting blood glucose levels. Even if you don't want to lose weight through mindful eating, you will still experience great health benefits, which makes it suitable for everyone.

The Importance of Mindful Eating

Current lifestyles constantly tempt people since food can be found anywhere and at any time. There are a myriad of other distractions constantly vying for attention, which makes it challenging to concentrate on one thing at a time. Consider what you usually do while you eat—scrolling through social media or your favorite TV show probably has a greater share of your attention than your meal. These distractions and behaviors create mindlessness, and over time, the act becomes automatic.

The issue with mindless eating is that you do not recognize cues of fullness and continue to eat. It takes about 20 minutes for your body to realize it is full, so being engrossed in distractions means you are missing this message from your brain. By the time you accept that you are full, you have already consumed too much food and feel bloated or experience a heaviness in your stomach. This is the main concern with binge eating and can be detrimental if you are consuming junk food.

Mindful eating assists you in concentrating on the act of eating. It forces you to consider whether you need to eat or want to eat. It aids in differentiating between physical hunger and emotional eating. By increasing your awareness when eating, you identify triggers that cause your cravings and can avoid them through mindfulness. It may seem like a huge task at the moment, but there are many tools and techniques that can increase your awareness so that you becomc a successful mindful eater.

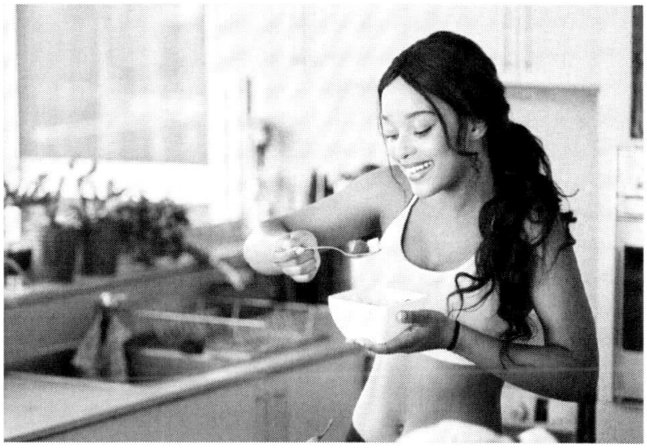

Mindful eating is so important that technologies exist to help you stay on the mindful track. Apps and trackers are a great tool to focus your mind on mindful eating, especially if you enjoy using technology. Search on your preferred app store for "mindful eating" and several options will appear that you might find useful. Select your favorite one and use it daily to support your efforts. These apps assist with determining why you want to eat, why you are hungry, work as food diaries, and encourage good decision-making. Some of these apps track your emotions and provide you with additional mindfulness exercises to enhance your awareness.

Characteristics of Mindful Eating

Mindful eating requires awareness or being fully present in the moment to work. This awareness is indicated through the following four characteristics:

- Remaining aware of your actions and how it affects your body, regardless of whether the effects are positive or negative.
- Using your senses to choose nutritious foods that provide a pleasant eating experience.
- Appreciating sensory responses to food without judgment.
- Being aware of how you feel, physical hunger, and fullness.

Mindful Eating Questionnaire

It is challenging to know exactly how aware you are if you do not have something to measure your mindfulness. A diverse group of researchers created a Mindful Eating Questionnaire, which is a scale to assist in determining mindfulness when eating. This scale consists of five factors with 28 items in total. Each part of the questionnaire is described below with details about the five factors.

Factor 1: Disinhibition

Disinhibition refers to a lack of self-control when it comes to matters of social norms. It manifests as poor decision-making and impulsivity, which may be due to cognitive or perceptual awareness issues. If you struggle to control your eating, then you might have disinhibition challenges. Some examples from the questionnaire include:

- Overeating when you attend an "all you can eat" buffet.
- Taking a second helping of food when you feel full.
- Upsizing (getting larger) meals if they don't cost too much, even when you don't feel really hungry.

Factor 2: Awareness

Awareness is all about being present in the moment and noticing small details. Eating food rapidly and mindless eating usually decreases your awareness and could be a sign that you are not paying attention to eating. Some elements from the questionnaire that show heightened awareness include:

- Appreciating the arrangement of food on a plate including colors, smells, and textures.
- Noticing subtle flavors while eating.
- Noticing how eating affects your emotional state.

Factor 3: External Cues

External cues are anything that prompts you to eat. For example, smelling a neighbor's barbeque leaves your mouth salivating or a promotion on your favorite fizzy drink makes you want to buy it. External cues are a major factor that you need to be aware of if you want to be a mindful eater. The questionnaire considers the following points, among others:

- Taking notice of food advertisements that create cravings.
- Notice when you feel sluggish after eating a large meal.
- Realizing you want to eat more than you should when attending events with good food.

Factor 4: Emotional Response

An emotional response is any feelings you experience. If you are an emotional eater, then this is the factor you should focus your energy on. Scale items regarding emotions include:

- Eating to feel better when you are sad.
- Difficulty staying away from sweet treats when they are in the house.
- Finding a snack to eat when you feel stressed.

Factor 5: Distraction

Distraction refers to not paying attention because something else is taking the spotlight. You become distracted whenever you are doing another activity while eating, even if you think it is something harmless like watching TV. The main points for this factor are:

- Wandering thoughts while eating.
- Thinking about your to-do list while eating.
- Eating food so quickly that you do not notice the taste.

Prepare To Be a Mindful Eater

Eating is complex—there are a ton of things to consider from what you should eat to when, not to mention determining whether you are experiencing emotional or physical hunger. There is so much conflicting information about diets that makes it challenging for you to know what is best. Luckily, mindful eating is a lifestyle that encourages awareness, rather than having strict rules about foods you can and cannot eat. Spend some time on your own, free from other distractions, and consider your current eating patterns and how you would like the situation to change. Think about how mindful eating plays a role in your future and the ways it could be beneficial to you. Now is the time to start setting goals for your mindful journey.

Chapter 4: Benefits of Mindful Eating

Mindful eating changes your behavior and enables you to experience your health in a better light. It is a great tool for a busy lifestyle and helps you to enjoy food while providing nutritional value to your body. Although the benefits to overeaters, emotional eaters, and binge eaters are clear, it is also beneficial to anyone else who has bad eating habits.

Body Benefits

Mindful eating has many advantages for your body. It gives you an opportunity to improve all parts of yourself. Not only will you see physical improvements, your body and organs will also thank you for looking after them better.

Better Digestion and Nutrient Absorption

When you eat quickly or do not chew food properly, you are swallowing large chunks of food. The intestine cannot absorb nutrients from larger food particles as the passages of the small intestine are tiny. Sometimes, the intestines don't absorb any nutrients because it has insufficient energy to digest food, which limits the abilities of your body. Mindful eating changes this situation. One of the ways you become more aware of eating is by chewing food thoroughly, which means you are eating slower. By breaking down your food, you help your body to digest food more easily. It also improves nutrient absorption, so your body gets a lot more goodness.

Enhanced Mind-Gut Communication

Practicing mindful eating strengthens the communication between your mind and your stomach. Once you have a strong communication system, you can understand what your body is trying to say more easily. As you start to identify your cravings as other bodily cues, you set yourself free from food cravings and concentrate on addressing the real concerns. You are not ignoring cravings as you would with a traditional diet. You acknowledge cravings as a symptom of another problem. A stronger connection between mind and gut also helps you realize when you are physically hungry and when you have had enough to eat.

Overall Health Improves

Your overall health will improve greatly if you become a mindful eater. Although it won't solve all your health problems, you will feel better, be more energized, and struggle less with digestive issues. Studies also found links between mindful eating and lower cholesterol and blood pressure levels. You may feel less stressed and anxious, which allows you to eat and sleep better. Mindful eating decreases cortisol levels too, which is the hormone that contributes to obesity. Blood sugar levels become easier to control and your cardiovascular health improves, so your chances of type 2 diabetes and heart problems decrease.

Overcoming Food Battles

You are probably reading this book because you are fighting some kind of food battle. There are so many different eating disorders and weight issues that you may suffer from, and mindful eating can help you address these problems. Having a better relationship with food is the ultimate benefit you derive from mindful eating.

Improves Weight Loss

Mindful eating may help you to lose weight. We have already looked at some research studies that support weight loss, and it is clear that alongside other health benefits of mindful eating, you could drop a few pounds in the long term. With mindful eating, you consider several questions before eating and immerse yourself in the experience. You will find you eat fewer calories, avoid impulsive eating, and choose healthier food options. It might take some getting used to, but you will succeed if you keep working hard. After a while, mindful eating will become entrenched in your lifestyle.

Addresses Eating Disorders

Mindful eating can help you overcome eating disorders by perceiving yourself and food in better ways. Previous research showed that binge eating decreases if you become a mindful eater as it improves self-control. Other eating disorders improve with mindfulness too, since you use various techniques to deal with your emotions, eating problems (including certain eating disorders), and depression.

Fewer Food Cravings

Mindful eating makes you more alert to your body's signals regarding hunger. You might realize that cues to eat are based on boredom, emotion, or peer pressure rather than physical hunger. Being able to distinguish between these different signals means you can alter your response and do not have to eat when you get a craving. Mindful eating enables you to take control of cravings and turn them into other cues which helps you to eat less.

Reduces Overeating

Eating mindfully means eating slowly. Taking longer to eat allows your stomach to send satiation cues to your brain before you can overindulge. It allows you to enjoy your food while making a conscious effort to eat healthier. Your body only sends fullness cues after 20 minutes, so how much would you normally eat in 20 minutes while watching TV? You might be able to finish a large helping of lasagna, a glass of soda, and a chocolate bar. In contrast, eating mindfully results in only eating half of the lasagna and a few sips of soda before you feel full. Leaving the rest of the lasagna and the chocolate bar greatly decreases the amount of food you eat. You might still enjoy the chocolate sometime, but it could be a fun-size bar every few days.

Fewer Food Hangovers

Overeating may cause "food hangovers," depending on the amount and type of food. Eating too quickly results in your stomach filling up faster than it can send satiation signals to your brain. Overeating leads to digestive upsets and may provide substantial amounts of energy before causing an energy dip. Your body requires substantial energy to digest food, so all your energy goes to digestion, which is why you experience fatigue shortly after eating. Mindful eating reduces the number of food hangovers you experience if you follow the basic principles.

Mental Health Benefits

You already know that the satisfaction you experience when eating food comes from a release of feel-good hormones. Mindful eating still allows for the release of these hormones, but this lifestyle encourages other ways to trigger hormones than just with food. You will gain many mental and emotional benefits from practicing mindfulness.

Increased Emotional Control

Emotions and eating have a lot to do with each other even if you aren't an emotional eater. You might restrict your food intake and feel down about it or you could be overeating when your emotions are unstable. Mindful eating teaches you to identify your emotions and deal with them in a productive manner. You will no longer eat your emotions. You will use food as a positive nutritional experience.

Alternative Stress-Busting Options

Emotional eating usually happens when a person experiences stress or feels upset. The problem is that emotional eating is seen as a weakness instead of a coping mechanism, but there are many other ways you might cope with stress. Some of these methods like exercising or meditating are good ways to deal with stress. In contrast, other methods such as excessive drinking and smoking are perceived as poor stress coping techniques. Mindful eating encourages you to deal with your emotions in healthy ways rather than through overeating. By understanding your emotions, you can identify stress triggers which helps you to find suitable stress-busting methods.

Stops The Fight

It might seem like you are constantly in a battle of wills when it comes to food. You think about what you should and shouldn't eat and wonder how some people can leave half a slice of cake on their plate when you finished yours a few minutes ago. These struggles take up time and energy, but it doesn't get you closer to your weight management goals. A preoccupation with food leads to feelings of guilt if you eat something you think is off-limits, and food restriction only increases cravings. With mindful eating, you consider food in a healthy manner and don't place limits on your food selection. This ability stops your internal battle between eating and emotions.

Building Trust

Why do you usually opt for a diet? You might feel that you cannot control your own eating patterns or that you need strict dietary guidelines. But, the truth is that you don't trust your own food decisions. Mindful eating does not give you a strict guideline about what you should or shouldn't consume, or when you must eat. Rather, mindful eating teaches you how to trust yourself, your mind, and your body's cues, because only you can fully understand your body and circumstances. Once you trust yourself, you gain the power to change your life.

Being Kind

Sometimes, you might look at yourself in the mirror and think you hate your body. You might have feelings of guilt or hatred towards yourself after emotional or binge eating. These negative thoughts will not create change. You cannot beat yourself up with hatred and expect that you will change overnight. Mindful eating allows you to accept yourself at every stage of the eating process and throughout your weight management journey. It encourages you to be aware of your good aspects while focusing on positive gains made through mindful eating practices. You will learn to be kind to yourself and actively seek out positivity for motivation when you face new obstacles.

Food-Related Benefits

The big problem with diets, whether to lose or put on weight, is that they restrict your food intake, and you can only select items from a limited food menu. Mindful eating doesn't have these restrictions at all. It allows you to eat what you want by considering your options and the effect on your body carefully. The benefits of variety and enjoying food are ones you don't easily find elsewhere.

Embracing the Middle Ground

If you have an "all or nothing" mentality, then it could be an obstacle to weight management. You might think you should eat no starches, no sugar, and no processed foods. Although these changes could be beneficial, it is not helpful for your mind or your weight management journey. You might find that you can stick with these restrictions for a few days or weeks, but once you are faced with these foods, you start to binge eat. Mindful eating will help you find the middle ground by allowing you to eat any food you want, within moderation, and through conscious decision-making.

Better-Tasting Food

Mindful eating requires you to concentrate on the eating process and the food you are consuming. When you have this intense focus, you start to re-experience food and appreciate the different flavors, textures, and scents. Through experiential eating, you discover new taste sensations that you might not have realized previously, even if it is a dish you ate frequently. Mindfulness allows you to enjoy food without feelings of guilt.

Greater Variety

Mindful eating tends to diversify your palate, and help you become open to trying new foods. You may find that your new awareness prickles your senses and you want to test a portion of food after seeing, smelling, or touching it. Allow yourself enough time to experience each food or ingredient fully by using all your senses, then decide whether you like it or not. Try new foods several times and on different occasions to ensure you give them a proper chance. You might find that your tastes change substantially, especially when you can incorporate more foods into your weekly menu.

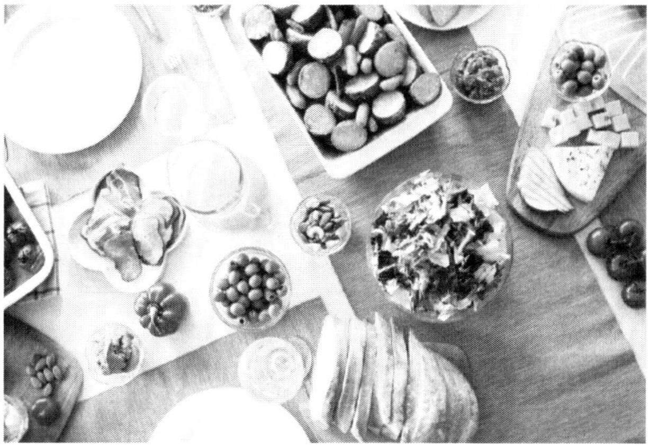

Efficacy of Mindful Eating

Mindfulness is a therapeutic practice that enables you to manage your eating habits better. The strategies used in mindfulness are quite diverse, which allows you to find methods that work for you based on your eating problems.

A Perpetual Loop

Any bad food habit or eating disorder creates a self-perpetuating loop. You feel upset about something, so you binge, eat your feelings, or avoid food altogether. After your eating behavior, you feel bad about your consumption decision which might result in eating again. This loop repeats itself over and over again. During this time, you are passing judgment on yourself.

Mindfulness focuses your attention on remaining in the moment. You start to identify elements within the current situation without any form of prejudice. Mindfulness alters your mindset and enables you to determine the best strategy to overcome challenges and move forward through positive change. In essence, mindful eating will break the perpetual loop by addressing your emotions, and help you to make better food decisions. Breaking this link requires a continuous focus on your end goal so that you stay the course.

Engaging the Prefrontal Cortex

The prefrontal cortex is a part of the brain. It is situated at the front of the brain and responsible for rational thinking. When you practice mindfulness techniques, especially meditation, you strengthen your prefrontal cortex, which means you think more rationally. A strong prefrontal cortex enables you to observe thoughts about food and be around food without acting on these impulses. Rational thinking promoted by mindfulness makes it easier to break bad habits and encourages the development of good habits.

It's Time for Action

There are so many benefits to mindful eating that it only makes sense to give it a try. Mindful eating nourishes the body, mind, and soul. By taking care of your body, you strengthen your mind and regain emotional control. You start to enjoy food in new ways, as you use all your senses and diversify your tastes. The best part is that you can still eat what you want as long as you remain mindful of your choices. The benefits are clear, and now is as good a time as ever to become a mindful eater.

Chapter 5: Principles of Mindful Eating

Mindful eating is something that you have to learn to do. You might be practicing some techniques already, which is great. Understanding the principles and theory of mindful eating can provide you with more techniques to improve your mindfulness skills. Over time, you will become more mindful and your eating habits will change, which makes you a healthier individual.

The basic principles of mindful eating are quite simple:

- Listen to your body's cues regarding hunger and satiety.
- Avoid overconsumption—eat anything you want in moderation.
- Deal with external cues effectively, such as eating smaller portions and eliminating distractions.

These three principles affect every part of mindful eating. Although the principles are few, they are great in-depth. Almost all other aspects of mindful eating can fall under one of these three principles. Many tools, models, and techniques exist to help you implement and maintain each of these principles.

The Mindful Eating Cycle

Mindful eating can be understood through a cycle of questions. These questions prompt the thinking process and help you recognize different eating behaviors. Together, these questions are called the mindful eating cycle, which was created by Doctor Michelle May. It considers six main questions: Why, when, what, how, how much, and where. Let's break these six topics down further.

Why

The first question is all about why you eat. Think about whether you are aware of situational and emotional triggers that make you want to eat, even when you aren't hungry. Consider the reasons why you eat when you made the decision not to eat. Evaluate previous diet attempts and determine which ones worked or why you didn't stick to the plan.

When

The next question considers when you eat. Take a moment to think about when you usually eat or drink something and why you decide to eat at these times. Reflect on whether you are hungry at these times and whether you can distinguish between physical and mental hunger. Think about other things you can do to redirect your attention instead of choosing food. Consider strategies to help you cope better when you experience an eating trigger. Think about whether your eating cues actually mean your body is trying to tell you something else.

What

Next, reflect on what you eat. Think about your food choices on a typical day, and consider using a food journal to help you identify eating patterns. Reflect on what foods you eat for different types of emotions and why you select this specific item. Consider times when you restricted food, how it made you feel, and whether you binge later on. Think about how you feel when you eat certain foods, and if you are worried about overeating these items. Ponder how your choice of food affects your health, and identify areas that you could improve. Come up with some changes you can make immediately, and the food you require to make these alterations. Reflect on the possibility of eating anything you want while keeping moderation in mind.

How

The act of eating is the next topic to consider. Determine what you eat, whether it is a food you truly enjoy eating, or whether you eat rapidly without tasting properly. Compare how you eat in public with how you eat in private and identify aspects that you need to transfer from one dimension to the other. To fully evaluate how you eat, imagine you have to write a review about the last meal you had. If you cannot describe it properly, then your awareness needs some improvements.

How Much

The next question is all about the amount you eat. Think about how you know you have had enough food and how you feel when you finish eating. Compare your feelings after a meal with how you want to feel after eating. Reflect on whether you consume everything on the plate and how you decide to stop eating if you do not feel hungry. Identify emotions and other triggers that cause you to overeat and create an action plan to deal with those situations better in the future. Consider what you do when you eat too much and how it affects the next few hours.

Where

For this question, consider how you use the energy from the food you eat. Determine what you do after eating and if you use the energy for physical activity. Compare being physically active with watching TV or lounging around the house. Think about how you use your free time and whether it is productive for the amount you eat. Take a moment to reflect on exercise. Identify how you feel about exercise, whether specific exercise is more enjoyable for you, or if you use exercise as punishment when you ate something that you perceive as bad. Consider other ways of using your time like finding new hobbies or starting a healthy habit. Poinder your goals for your life and reflect on how you could use your energy to make these things happen. Determine your self-care routines and how you can incorporate wellness into your available time.

The mindful eating cycle allows you to consider your consumption habits as part of a whole, rather than simply identifying it as a problem. This cycle runs continuously so you can start thinking about any question. Whenever you want to eat or think about food, come back to these ideas. It can help you to identify eating challenges and allows you to build a healthy relationship with food.

The Essence of Mindful Eating

Mindful eating allows you to find the middle ground between restrictive eating and eating mindlessly. To do this requires a lot of self-control and self-belief. You can get results if you continue to be mindful. It might seem a bit vague now, but once you start practicing mindfulness, you will quickly adjust to a new way of thinking about food. Follow the next few ideas about mindful eating to help you in your efforts.

The Food Relationship is Permanent

Food is necessary for survival and it will always be a fixture in your life. Your relationship with food may shift from positive to negative and everything in between, but you cannot ignore it. Start to see food for what it is, something to be enjoyed and nourishing for your body.

You Know Your Mental and Physical Needs

You are the only one who knows what you need. You know the needs of your body and your mind. Nobody else knows what your true needs are and they cannot fully understand your body. If you go to a restaurant with friends, they cannot eat your food for you and they cannot decide when you are full because only you can eat for your own body and know when your body cues indicate fullness. The same goes for diets and portion suggestions. These are just a guide, they cannot determine when you have had enough, and they don't know when you are hungry. Start trusting that you know what your body needs by tuning in to its communication.

Your Thoughts and Feelings are a Source of Information

Your thoughts and feelings provide a myriad of information. They inform you about what your body or mind needs and prompt you to take action. If you have weight challenges, then you might find that your thoughts and feelings are negative. Sometimes, you even use your thoughts to punish yourself when you are something you perceived as wrong which causes you to feel bad about yourself. Mindful eating discourages negative thoughts and feelings—do not play into your negativity. Instead, acknowledge your thoughts or emotions, and use them as a guide to making a better decision about what you need.

Explore and Understand

Diets expect you to control yourself through willpower alone. Whenever a minor slip-up happens, you feel guilty, which results in struggling with your emotions and dissatisfaction. Willpower alone is unlikely to be effective, especially if you are on a restricted diet. Mindful eating rejects this concept. Instead, you use all eating experiences as an opportunity to explore different foods. Simultaneously, you learn to identify and understand your emotions, triggers, and cravings. You stop thinking in terms of good and bad and refocus on enjoyment and health.

No Bad Foods Exist

You can eat any food you want if you are a mindful eater. Absolutely no foods are off-limits. Accept that foods have different nutritional values and that one food may be more advantageous than another. Any food is acceptable when consumed in moderation, and you can do so without feeling guilty afterward. What does change is your experience when eating various foods which allows you to derive satisfaction from mindful eating.

Calories Count

Mindful eating does not require that you count calories, but you should still be aware of the calorie content of the foods you eat. Consider your budget for a moment. You don't necessarily keep track of every purchase, but you do have a good idea about average prices, when something is too expensive, or when you found a bargain. Calories in mindful eating are the same. You do not need to count calories, but calories do count. They are a meaningful way to remain aware.

Look at food labels to identify calorie values, or find the calories in fresh produce by doing an internet search. For example, the average apple weighs six ounces and contains approximately 88 calories; in contrast, three ounces of milk chocolate has 455 calories. What a big difference! In the future, you might choose apples when you have a craving for something sweet, or you could decide to eat a smaller amount of chocolate. Checking calorie counts makes it a lot easier to make healthy food choices and enjoy food sensibly.

Use Inner and Outer Wisdom

Inner wisdom comes from your thoughts, emotions, and experience. In contrast, outer wisdom is derived from external influences, such as a specific context, or cues from your surroundings. When you become a mindful eater, you become aware of how inner and outer wisdom works together for your own good. You might think about a birthday dinner you are attending later in the week (external wisdom), and decide to eat only healthy foods until then (internal wisdom), so that you can spoil yourself by enjoying a favorite. Your food and eating decisions will fluctuate, but you can use these two wisdoms to guide your choices.

Find Joy in Every Bite

Mindfulness urges you to stay in the moment and enjoy what you are doing. Everything you do is an experience and you can learn something from it. Mindful techniques help to focus your mind on what you are doing which enhances your experience. As you choose your food and with every bite, you use your senses. You might find yourself identifying with a new taste, texture, or scent. Besides providing nutrients for your body, you also feed your soul through experiential, mindful eating.

Life Doesn't Revolve Around Food

For some people, food is the be-all and end-all. If you are one of these people, then you cannot think about a life or event without food. This obsession with food will decrease as you improve your mindful eating skills. Eating is just one small part of your life and you need to find a balance between eating and other activities. You are in control of your life and you can effect change when you realize there is a lot more to life than only food. You will start to explore new activities, practice hobbies, and become more mindful in general once your relationship with food improves. Food is only part of the journey, so enjoy the rest of your life too.

Helpful Tools

There are many tools available to help you stay present in the moment and become more aware of your relationship with food. The ideas above provide some guidance when it comes to mindful eating. The next few ideas provide practical assistance if you prefer a hands-on approach.

The Hunger Scale

A scale can help you to determine the extent of your hunger, and help you decide whether you should be eating. The scale ranges from one to ten and describes several stages of hunger, as created by Eugenia Killoran. Whenever you feel like eating, pull out this scale, and find out just how hungry you are, or whether you are about to eat mindlessly.

1. **Ravenous**

You feel like you are starving. When you are ravenous you could experience feelings of weakness, be dizzy, or have a headache. You struggle to concentrate and have no energy.

2. **Uncomfortably Hungry**

You are cranky or irritable, combined with feelings of low energy and nausea.

3. **Very Hungry**

You have a strong urge to eat and your stomach feels empty of all food.

4. **A Little Hungry**

Your bodily cues plant thoughts of eating in your mind, and you start to consider when to eat.

5. **Neutral**

You have eaten sufficiently to have energy, and you feel satisfied psychologically and physically.

6. **Satisfied and Light**

Your body is satisfied with the amount you ate, but you still feel light.

7. **Full**

Although you are satisfied, you feel you still eat a bit more. Your body no longer needs food, but your mind urges you to eat more.

8. **Very Full**

You start to have a tummy ache from the amount you ate, The food tasted so good that you continued eating, even though you knew you had enough.

9. **Uncomfortably full**

You feel bloated, heavy, tired, and full to the point of discomfort.

10. **Painfully full**

A typical food coma. You have eaten way too much, like when you participate in a Thanksgiving or Christmas dinner. You are in great physical discomfort and avoid movement. You might consider never looking at food again.

The most comfortable hunger levels range from three to six. If you want to eat mindfully, then eat when you rate your hunger at level three. Stop eating as soon as you reach level six. Sticking to these scale points ensures you do not go hungry while preventing overeating.

Awareness Checklist

The awareness checklist ensures you are being mindful and enhances awareness when eating. It contains six questions, so keep a copy close by whenever you decide to eat.

1. Am I sitting down?
2. Am I eating slowly or fast?
3. Am I tasting each bite or eating mindlessly?
4. On a scale ranging from one to ten, how hungry am I?
5. Am I concentrating on only the food or engaged in multitasking?
6. Am I stressed, anxious, bored, or do I have a rumbling stomach?

Mindful Eating Checklist

Another great tool is a checklist for mindful eating. This checklist can be used to increase your awareness. It may take some time to get through this checklist initially, but it will become part of your daily life soon enough.

Meals

The checklist starts by considering meals.

During your meals, ensure that you:

- Pause between bites
- Become aware of the flavor(s)
- Become aware of the texture(s)
- Take deep breaths
- Put away digital devices

Consider the predominant textures while eating. Are they:

- Crunchy
- Creamy
- Dry
- Grainy
- Moist
- Something else?

Next, reflect on the main flavors or tastes. Are they:

- Salty
- Sweet
- Sour
- Bitter
- Umami (savory)

Snacks

When eating snacks, you should also be mindful. Much mindless eating occurs while snacking. You can improve your mindfulness while snacking by following this checklist:

- Take smaller bites
- Chew your food thoroughly
- Eat slowly

Recap

Once you finish your food, make some notes about the experience. You can make these notes beneath the checklist or use a food diary to keep track of what you are eating and the mindfulness experience.

Mindful Eating For Children

Children who are taught to be mindful eaters are more likely to have a healthy relationship with food as adults. You can start to teach your children about mindful eating from a young age, but still ensure they get the required nutrients for growth. Most of the strategies that encourage mindful eating children are similar to those used by adults. The important thing to remember is that your children are still learning to think rationally and will learn about food from you, so you have to set the example and guide your children.

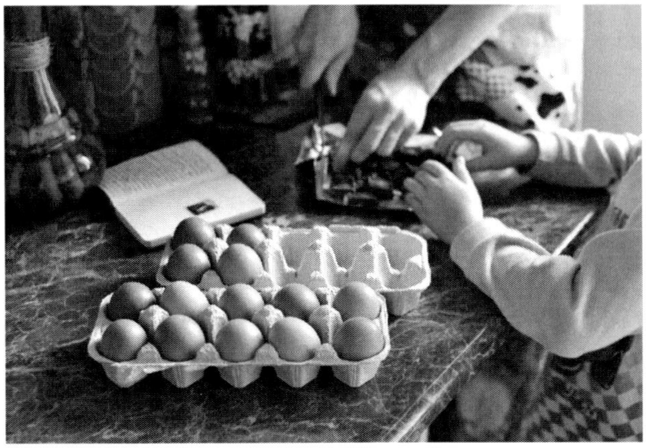

No Screens at The Table

If you visit any restaurant, then you will be amazed at the number of children staring at a phone or tablet screen while eating their food. This also happens during meal times at home, and you might be guilty of this offense too. Any type of screen, whether it be a phone, tablet, or television, will be a distraction at the dinner table. The same goes for smartwatches or radios blaring in the background as well. Teach your children to eat their food without staring at a screen. It will help them to learn more about the food in front of them, increase their enjoyment, and they will start to listen to their body's cues when they become full.

Eating Together

It is always best to eat meals at a table and as a family. When you eat together, you can watch how your children interact with their food and their likes and dislikes. It allows you to refocus their attention on food when they want to do something else and provides an opportunity to concentrate on your children.

Before your family starts eating, take a few moments to be thankful for the food, or let your children take a few deep breaths. This short quiet time allows your child to calm down and reduce distractions before paying attention to their meal.

Table Manners

Mindful eating requires awareness of everything to do with eating which includes teaching your children about table manners. Teach them how to use utensils properly and how to talk about food properly. Explain to your child that they need to take small bites and chew their food properly. One way to ensure this happens is to ask your child to put down their utensils between bites. Encourage them to excuse themselves from the table properly, and make them responsible for cleaning up any spills they make to make them aware of wastage.

Talk About the Food

Chatting to your children about food is a great way to increase their awareness. You can use the mindful eating checklist and ask your children the same questions reflected on it. Ask them to explain what the food looks like, the taste, and how it feels. With smaller children, and when introducing new foods, you could let your child pick up the food with their hands to fully immerse themself in the experience.

Ask your child about how their belly feels before, during, and after eating. You could also ask how hungry your child feels before they start eating. This makes your child aware of their body's cues and helps them identify feelings of fullness. You could also let your child serve their own food (with your assistance), and guide them in their portion sizes. However, do not force them to eat everything on the plate if they say they are full. Trust that your child knows their body. They will come to ask you for food if they are truly hungry, and you can then help them determine if they are really hungry or just bored. If your child asks for seconds or says they are hungry soon after meals, then tell them they have to wait 15 minutes, and then ask if they still want something to eat. It gives the stomach and brain time to communicate with each other and your child will start doing something else if the cravings are driven by boredom.

Don't Eat on the Go

Do not allow your children to eat while you are in the car or in a rush. Eating on the go will teach your children that it is okay to multitask while eating, makes food a cure for boredom, and will make them less aware of the eating process. If you are worried that your child will go hungry, then take a few moments to sit on a bench and eat something before you go about your tasks. This encourages your child to make time for food and increases awareness of mindful eating.

Ready for Mindful Eating

Mindful eating is possible if you put in the time and effort to be aware continuously. The principles of mindful eating are easy to remember, so make a note of them and keep this note handy whenever you have doubts. There are many guidelines to improve your mindfulness and tools to help you remain mindful. Try out one or all of these techniques and identify which ones work best for you. It will take time to get into the swing of things, so be patient with yourself. Over time, you will see the advantages of mindful eating, and find it easier to incorporate it into daily life.

Chapter 6: Make Mindful Eating a Habit

Mindful eating only becomes a habit if you continuously concentrate on being aware and never give up on the process. The benefits of mindful eating far outweigh the time and effort it takes to turn it into a habit. After a while, mindful eating will become second nature to you and your hard work will reap rewards.

Mindful Eating Activities

Several activities and exercises can help you become more mindful. All of these activities work by focusing on specific aspects of the food in front of you. Through these exercises, you learn to appreciate food and your relationship with food improves greatly.

The Food Critic

Mindful eating might seem strange, but there is an easy way to improve mindfulness, be a food critic. A food critic is a professional judge of a plate of food made by someone. Most food critics dine at luxury restaurants or up-and-coming food establishments, but there are also other places for food critics. Think about some of the reality TV shows, such as Masterchef, where judges evaluate contestants' food or a local carnival where there is a competition for the best food. All of these events have someone who is judging.

You can pretend you are a food critic, and "judge" the food. When you take on the role of a food critic, you automatically pay closer attention to the food, the appearance, smell, and taste. Always have a positive attitude when judging food. Make notes of what you enjoyed about the food and what you would like to try again. This is a helpful technique if you are trying out new food, or when you are uncertain about the dish in front of you. It is a useful exercise, because it will help you identify foods that work well together, or when a dish needs another element, like seasoning or sauce, to help it improve. This activity is easy to do with children as well and will help them cultivate a love for mindful eating.

The Raisin Meditation

A prolific mindful eating exercise comes from Jon Kabat Zinn, a mindfulness expert. Zinn created an exercise to increase your awareness while eating by using a single raisin. It works wonders for mindfulness and helps you to focus on nothing else at that moment. Once you have done this exercise, you can also try it with other foods, if you want some extra practice.

Follow these instructions for the raisin meditation:

1. **Hold**

Pick up the raisin and hold it between your index finger and thumb or place it in the palm of your hand.

2. **See**

Pay close attention to how the raisin looks. One way to do this is to imagine you have never seen a raisin before and you want to examine this strange object. Gaze over every part of the raisin. Concentrate your attention on the folds of the raisin. Focus on the ridges that cast off light, and then move on to the hollows that are darker in color. Try to find asymmetrical lines or unique patterns on the surface of the raisin.

3. **Touch**

Use your fingers to turn the raisin around and explore the texture. You can either turn it around on your palm, or pick it up and turn it in your fingers. Try touching the raisin with different fingers to see how the texture changes. Sometimes, it helps to close your eyes when doing this step as it may increase your sense of touch.

4. **Smell**

Bring the raisin to your nose, and inhale deeply. Try to describe the aroma or fragrance of the raisin. Take several breaths to fully enjoy the smell. Take note of any changes in your mouth or stomach while doing this step.

5. **Place**

Bring the raisin to your lips slowly while noticing the position of your hand and arm. Take a moment to appreciate that your hand knows the exact position in front of your mouth. Open your mouth and place the raisin inside, but do not chew it. Feel the raisin with your tongue, and focus on the sensation your mouth creates from the raisin's presence.

6. **Taste**

Prepare to chew the raisin by positioning it in the right place in your mouth. Notice where the raisin is between your teeth so that you can chew it properly. With full consciousness, bite into the raisin once or twice. Take note of any tastes coming from the raisin. Continue to chew the raisin fully, but do not swallow it. Concentrate on how the taste and texture change as you chew, and how it feels in your mouth.

7. **Swallow**

Before you swallow the raisin, become fully aware of your body's actions. Try to identify the precise moment when your body has the intention to swallow so that you become hyper-aware. Swallow the raisin.

8. Follow

Attempt to trace the raisin down your throat and as it moves into your stomach. Focus your awareness on how your body feels during this exercise and after eating the raisin.

Utensil Play

Eating utensils, such as knives, forks, and spoons, are tools to help you get your food into your mouth. Your utensils can help you become more aware, because the way you hold and use these items may make you unattentive. Think about it this way—you probably eat popcorn with your hands since it is easier than trying to stab it with a fork or scoop it with a spoon. Although it makes it easier to eat popcorn with your hands, it requires less attention.

For this exercise, you are going to change the way you use your utensils. These activities are suitable for individuals of all ages, but children should be supervised, especially if you give them a knife. Use these steps to have a mindful eating experience:

Prepare Utensils and Food

Prepare a meal that you can eat with various utensils. For example, a salad or a pasta dish. Serve some of it on a plate and add some to a bowl. Gather up all your utensils, and place them on the table with the served food. You can use any utensils you want, but try to have at least a fork, knife, spoon, and chopsticks, or something similar. You can have utensils of different sizes or even odd choices such as toothpicks or plastic cutlery.

Use Your Normal Utensils

Select the utensils you would usually use for the dish in front of you and take a few bites from the plate and from the bowl. You might select a knife and fork if you are eating pasta from a plate, while a spoon could be easier if you are eating from a bowl. Use all your mindful techniques to be fully aware during the eating process. It might help you to have a piece of paper with you to make notes after each utensil about how you experienced the food.

Change the Position

Keep eating with your traditional utensils but change the position you are holding them in. This step works best with a fork. If the prongs of your fork point up, then you probably scoop the food, which is quite easy to do. Turn the fork the other way around, so that the prongs point towards the plate. You now need to get food by stabbing it and that requires precision. Stabbing food automatically makes you more aware, as the movements are controlled and require your full attention.

Utensil Swap

Try swapping your utensils to the other hand. Holding your utensils differently than usual automatically forces you to concentrate and be more aware since additional signals are sent between the hand and brain. If you are using a spoon, you might find that movements are not as controlled. Similarly, stabbing a tomato with a fork becomes more challenging while using a different hand.

Change Utensils

Use the different utensils you laid out to eat your food. Try eating salad with a spoon or a smaller fork. Smaller or challenging utensils increase your awareness because the movements must be precise if you want to get food to your mouth. Try changing to entirely different utensils. Chopsticks or toothpicks can be an interesting change and force you to pay attention.

Write down how you experience food while using different utensils. Make notes of the easiest and most challenging ones. Next time you struggle to eat mindfully, change your utensils to a challenging one so that your brain works harder. If you are eating too fast then choose a smaller utensil, which only allows you to take small bites at a time, and remember to put down your utensils between bites.

The Mindful Plate

Mindful eating allows you to enjoy food, improve your health, reduce negativity, and avoid unhealthy eating habits. There are many ways to achieve these ideals. Doctor Susan Albers uses a plate and glass to identify the key aspects of mindful eating. The plate is divided into four sections that help to improve your food relationship.

Plate Element 1: Observe

Whenever you want to eat, or while you are eating, observe how your mind and body respond to the situation. Notice what is happening with your body, such as having a rumbling stomach, feeling very hungry, or starting to feel full. Consider other physical sensations such as being tired, stressed, or having little energy.

Plate Element 2: Savor

Take note of different aspects of your meal. Determine the different aromas, flavors, and textures. Think about whether the food is hot or cold, sweet or salty, spicy or crunchy. Try to describe the taste as much as possible.

Plate Element 3: In-the-moment

Remain fully present throughout the entire eating experience. Remove any distractions, and sit down while you eat. Switch off electronic devices and concentrate only on the food.

Plate Element 4: Non-judgment

Be kind to yourself when you are eating and do not pass judgment. Mindful eating has no limitations. All you need to do is remain aware. Take note of any negative thoughts that rear their head and dismiss these thoughts while remembering that you are nourishing your body.

Glass: Awareness

The glass accompanying the plate signals awareness. It ties together all of the plate elements and summarizes what mindful eating is about. While you are eating, concentrate on how the food tastes and how it nourishes your body instead of mindlessly munching your food.

The mindful plate and glass analogy assists you in remaining aware during the eating process. It encourages you to consider every element of yourself and the food in front of you. By using these elements, you increase awareness of your mind, body, feelings, and thoughts. This technique is one of the easiest to do continuously and whenever you eat.

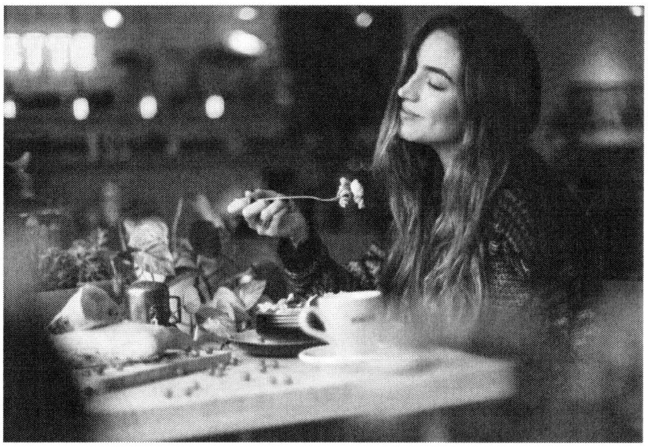

Two Plates

The two plates exercise is another useful tool to help you learn about mindful eating. It helps you to identify suitable portion sizes which is necessary if you think you might be overeating or have difficulty with identifying suitable portions. You can try this exercise at home to make mindful portioning easier. This approach is an excellent resource if you frequently dine out, when you think you have been served a too big portion, or when visiting all-you-can-eat buffets.

Here are the steps for the two plates technique:

1. **Get Two Plates**

Get two plates for you to use with your meal. One plate is a serving plate, while the other is an eating plate. If possible, use a smaller plate as your eating plate. Fill the serving plate with all the food you want to eat.

2. **Replate**

Move some of the food onto your eating plate from the serving plate. You can decide how much you want to place on the eating plate. Listen to cues from your body, and consider the amount you are most likely to eat. Try to figure out how hungry you are before you move food to the eating plate.

3. **Prepare the Food**

Use only the eating plate for this step. Cut all the food into bite-sized chunks. Prepare your food for eating in any other way, such as adding salad dressing or seasoning.

4. **Eat**

Start eating and concentrate on the food in front of you. Be mindful of every bite, and chew slowly. Only eat the food on your eating plate. You can finish all the food on this plate if you want to.

5. **Evaluate**

Once you have cleared your eating plate of food, evaluate how you feel. Determine if you are still hungry. Identify whether this is real hunger or whether you just want to eat more because the food tastes good. If you are no longer hungry, then you are done with your meal. If you still feel hungry, then move to the next step.

6. **Replate**

Move half of the food from your serving plate onto your eating plate. Repeat steps three and four with this serving. Cut up the food, and eat it mindfully.

7. **Evaluate**

Eat the food on your eating plate until you are full, or until you have cleared your plate. Reevaluate your hunger. Repeat steps six and seven, if you are still hungry. If you feel you are becoming full or think you have had enough, then you can push the remaining food aside and stop eating.

Mindful Eating Worksheet

The mindful eating worksheet is the perfect activity if you want to teach your children about this concept. It is suitable for all ages, so adults can enjoy this exercise too. Each section of the worksheet is outlined below, so you can use it to complete the exercise. Use your food diary or a loose page to gather all your ideas for the exercise in one place.

A Reminder

Start off by reminding yourself about the basics of mindful eating. You should be aware of how food tastes, feels, smells, and sounds.

The Experience

Choose a piece of fruit to eat mindfully. Eat the fruit, then make notes about your experience. Alternatively, make a drawing about your mindful experience.

Answer Questions

In the next section, you will answer questions about your experience. You can either think back to the experience while eating the fruit or you can eat something else, and then answer the questions.

- How did it taste?
- How did it look?
- How did it smell?
- How did it feel?
- How did it sound?

After considering each sense, answer this question: What did I notice about this food that I have not noticed before?

Expression

The final part of the worksheet is a space for expression and reflection. Spend some time drawing a picture of the fruit or other food, and draw everything you think it needs to grow. You can include drawings of people, machines, natural conditions, or anything else.

Tips and Strategies

Mindful eating needs to become a habit if you want to make it part of your lifestyle. There are numerous ways to incorporate it into daily life. Some of these changes are small and easy to implement while others may take a bit more time.

Plan and Prepare

Planning and preparing to eat mindfully is one of the first things you will do during this process. Spend sufficient time on preparing yourself mentally and getting the things you need to make a success of mindful eating.

- Eat one meal mindfully each day for a week, then add more mindful meals.
- Schedule time to eat into your diary and do not multitask at all when eating.
- Check food labels and calorie content of different foods frequently so that you can make sensible choices.
- If you want to eat calorie-dense foods, then choose a smaller portion and use it as a special treat. Most importantly, eat these foods mindfully and do not feel guilty about it afterward—it was a conscious decision.
- Sit down when you are ready to eat and switch off any distractions.
- Take a moment to feel thankful for the food you have before you start to eat. Look at each item specifically and name it. Consider the time and effort that went into growing the individual ingredients and making the meal.
- Measure your hunger level before you eat something, especially if it is a snack. It might be stress driving you to eat which requires other strategies than food.

When Eating

- Start eating when you feel only a bit hungry since extreme hunger will make you eat food impulsively.
- Only dish up a portion that you believe you can eat mindfully. Remember, it is about quality eating rather than the quantity you eat. You can always go back for a bit more later if you still feel physical hunger.
- Take small bites and chew your food slowly. Put down your fork in between bites, and only pick it up once you have swallowed the previous bite.
- Chew each bite about 30 times, although some foods could require more chewing and others less.

- Ensure that your meal takes at least 20 minutes to eat.
- Never eat from the packaging. Always serve your food on a plate or in a bowl.
- Don't force yourself to eat every bite on your plate. It is okay to stop eating once you are full.

Increase Awareness

- Concentrate on the smell, shape, texture, and taste of your food. Use the first few bites of each meal to emphasize each of these senses.
- Eat a variety of foods including those you would not normally try. For example, choose plant-based proteins instead of animal proteins. Consume any new foods mindfully so that you can experience them fully.
- Use a food diary to keep track of what you eat if this something you think could be valuable to you. Write down how hungry you are and how you are feeling before each meal. Make notes of how your mindful eating experience went and how you feel after eating.
- If your mind wanders while eating, acknowledge the thought and let it pass by, then continue with mindful eating on your next bite.
- Take note of how your first bite tasted versus the fifth and the last bite.

In the Kitchen

- Keep surface areas free of clutter and food. If you can see food, you are more likely to eat it, so pack all food into organized cupboards.
- Make healthy snacks easy to get. Cut fresh vegetables and fruit into smaller pieces and place them in small containers. Eat the contents of one of these packs when you feel slightly hungry.
- Avoid purchasing extra food and limit the amount of processed, refined foods in your home.
- Ensure that smaller plates and bowls are easy to reach—it makes it easier to serve smaller portions.
- Have a shopping list handy to write down any favorite healthy foods so you don't run out of these options.

You Can Do It

Mindful eating is possible. All you need to do is to start. Make a decision today to work hard on becoming a mindful eater. It helps to identify a few easier changes, and focus your energy on doing them fully. Once you master smaller changes, incorporate more difficult alterations into your life. Write out the tips and techniques that can help you best and put them up in the kitchen and dining room to assist you in maintaining mindfulness. Over time, you will find that mindful eating becomes second nature and even things you once thought challenging become easier.

Chapter 7: Coping Strategies Instead of Eating

Deciding to change your eating habits is a huge undertaking. It requires dedication, perseverance, and hard work. Although healthy eating is a noble cause, there is an obstacle. Most problematic eating stems from emotional issues, such as stress, depression, boredom, or frustration. If you do not address these issues, then your healthy eating efforts will be in vain. You risk slipping back into old habits or might pick up new bad habits, such as smoking. The best way to deal with this situation is to cope with your personal and emotional problems in a healthy manner.

Mindful eating has its roots in mindfulness, which alludes to the fact that you should have a heightened awareness of everything you do. Applying mindfulness to your life will help you overcome bad habits for good. Mindfulness also helps you to develop better coping strategies for problematic behaviors. By channeling your energy into productive activities, you learn to deal with personal problems and set the scene for successful mindful eating.

Mindfulness

You already know how to be a mindful eater, so now is your chance to bring this concept into other areas of your life. Mindfulness requires constant attention, and you will need some practice to make it a habit. The basic premise of mindfulness is to become more aware of the things around you and your place within a specific context. It allows you to experience things with all your senses.

Here is a quick mindfulness exercise for you to try by becoming aware of your current surroundings. Set a timer for two minutes. Take a look at the room around you and decide to focus on a specific object. Name the object, then look to the right of the object, and name the next object you see. Continue to do this for the full two minutes. All you want to do is to name what you are seeing, but do so without judgment. Once your two minutes are up, determine how you feel about the room. Identify something you didn't realize was in the room or that you sometimes look over such as a painting that has been on the wall for years. Focus on this object for a few seconds and take it in properly. This simple exercise has made you more aware of the things around you.

Mindfulness can be done internally to help you identify emotions and understand yourself properly. When you get up in the morning, take a moment to identify your current emotions, energy level, and thoughts. Do not pass judgment during the process; only observe these feelings and thoughts, then let them go. Repeat this process before lunch and before going to bed. You can repeat this exercise at any time during the day as it can help you to calm down when everything seems frantic.

Meditation

Meditation is a form of mindfulness because it requires you to stay still while observing the current moment. You can obtain guided meditations through videos and sound clips or you can read up on them and follow the steps by yourself. There are various types of meditations that take from a few minutes to an hour or more. Find the ones that work best for you and use them frequently to help you overcome emotional eating. Commit to meditating for about five minutes a day, and then bump it up to longer periods once you are ready. Below are a few meditation exercises for you to try.

Several studies have proven there are benefits to mindfulness and meditation. One study done in 2013 indicated that mindfulness meditation practiced consistently over eight weeks resulted in lower physical and mental stress, which assisted in decreasing stress-related inflammation and irritable bowel syndrome. Another study found that pain, anxiety, and depression decreases over a one-year period of meditation in individuals with chronic pain. Furthermore, meditations reduce generalized anxiety while improving self-confidence, since participants focus more on positive affirmations and self-love. Additional studies indicate that meditating for as little as minutes per day enhances memory and attention span within eight weeks (Basso et al., 2019; Hoge, et al., 2013; Rosenkranz et al., 2013). With all these benefits, it is no wonder that meditation is an excellent tool to assist with weight issues that frequently accompany stress, anxiety, depression, and other emotional or mental health issues.

Breathing Awareness Meditation

With this meditation, you will be concentrating on your breathing. It allows you to focus on only one thing, which improves your general awareness in other activities. It also helps you to calm down, improves concentration, and relieves anxiety.

1. Take slow deep breaths.
2. Focus on how the air expands your chest as you inhale through your nose, and how it collapses as you exhale through your mouth.
3. It could help you to count as you inhale and exhale, but do not let this distract you from your breathing concentration.
4. Acknowledge any thoughts that pop into your head and then set them free as if they are mist moving through air. Only focus on your breathing.

Loving Kindness Meditation

The aim of this meditation is to help you develop a sense of self-love. It helps you to be kind to yourself, other people, and stimuli that may cause stress.

1. Take a few deep breaths.
2. Open your mind to receive love and kindness.
3. Send mental messages of love and kindness to yourself and the outside world.

Relaxation Meditation

This meditation is fantastic if you need to set yourself free of tension or relieve stress. Your body can hold a lot of tension and you might not even realize it. Tense shoulders, cramping limbs, or muscle aches can be due to stress and emotional issues. Relaxing through meditation will help you to cope with your emotions and prevent you from reaching for food.

1. Lie flat on your back or sit comfortably in a chair. Keep your posture open and do not cross your arms or legs over each other. Keep them at your sides.
2. Close your eyes and take a few deep breaths.
3. Focus on relaxing your toes for a few seconds by clenching your muscles together and then releasing them. Continue with this clenching and release movement through all muscle groups in your body. Relax both feet, and release tension from your ankles.
4. Relax your calves fully, then your knees and your thighs. Spend enough time on these areas as you can have built-up tension in them.
5. Concentrate on relaxing your pelvic bone and hips, and feel them melting into the floor as all tension is released. Scrunch your buttocks together and release this position.
6. Release tension in your abdomen and lower back, then in your upper back and chest.
7. Allow your fingers to relax by clenching then releasing, moving up to your wrists, forearms, elbows, and upper arms.
8. Scrunch your shoulders upwards. Relax your shoulders fully and ensure that you are not pulling them up or holding excess tension. Let it all go. Relax your neck muscles.
9. Purse your lips together and then release them into a neutral position to remove tension. Scrunch your face muscles and release them, then do the same with your eyes. Crease your forehead into a frown, then relax completely.
10. Continue to take deep breaths as you relax fully. Open your eyes when you are ready.

Kindness Meditation

Being kind to yourself is something you should do all the time. It is difficult to look at yourself kindly if you feel your eating habits are poor or when a craving becomes intense. Use this meditation to help you overcome feelings of negativity and to improve your kindness towards your body and soul.

1. Sit down in a quiet and comfortable area such as a favorite couch, in the garden, or on some pillows.
2. Close your eyes and turn your attention to your breathing. Notice how the air moves through your body and the rise and fall of your chest. Become aware of the present moment.
3. Ask your breath to be a messenger as it moves through your entire body and mind. Let it communicate how you are feeling at this moment. Notice the message, but do not judge or react to it.
4. Tune into your breathing again. Find the pause right before you exhale. Feel the negativity and tension leaving your body as you exhale.
5. Visualize a loving presence. It could be someone you feel loved by, someone who has passed away, a beloved friend, or a spiritual figure. It could even be an animal or an inanimate object. The loving presence should bring about feelings of peace, safety, and love.

6. Focus on the loving feelings this presence imparts on you. Feel it warming you from the inside out, or imagine being hugged by this presence allowing the light to penetrate from the outside inward. Allow all these feelings and positive emotions to be with you in the moment.
7. Let the presence speak affirmations to you, such as saying "You are beautiful," "I love you," or "You make a difference." Don't force this communication, just think about what the person might say to you to help you experience positive vibrations.
8. Put your hand over your heart. Press these enlightening emotions into your body, allowing them to seep through your body and penetrate every cell. Continuously repeat the positive affirmations.
9. Place your arms around your body to embrace yourself in a hug. You could use other physical touches to help you experience the presence too such as stroking your hair, patting yourself on the shoulder, or touching your cheek. Allow yourself to be surrounded by love and light. Let it emerge from your core and radiate from your body.
10. Spend some time in this joyous moment. Once you are ready, slowly open your eyes, and continue your day with this focus on kindness.

Journal

Journaling is a simple mindfulness practice and emotional coping tool. It requires you to write down your thoughts and feelings, which will help you understand yourself better. Many people find that writing assists them in identifying troublesome behaviors, triggers, or deep-rooted emotional issues that require professional help. Identifying emotional problems allows you to work through your thoughts and emotions in a productive manner. Use a dedicated journal for emotional eating. You could even use the same one used as a food diary.

Start the journaling process by writing down your current state, what you are happy about, and any unhappiness. Pay special attention to your feelings and relationships towards food. Your journal is a space for honesty, so write down your true feelings. Do not try to sugarcoat the truth. Repeat this journaling exercise once a week and see how your perspective changes.

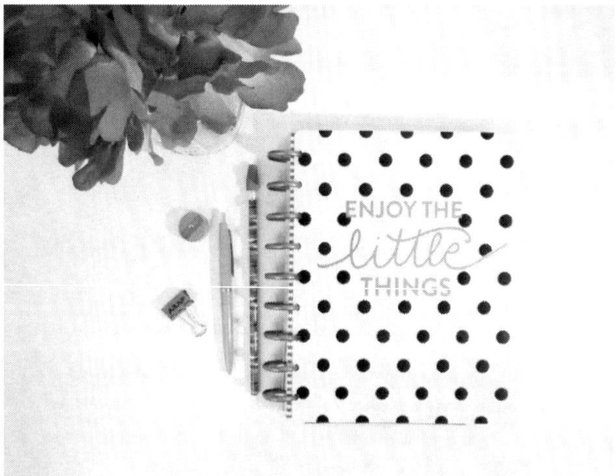

Journaling daily is the best way to deal with fluctuating emotions. Make some notes in the morning, before and after meals, and before you go to sleep about your current emotional state, and how it affects your eating. Journal prompts are useful if you do not know what to write about. A prompt is a statement or question that gives you inspiration for your writing. Try some of the following prompts to help you with mindful eating and general mindfulness.

- How hungry are you?
- How do you feel while eating?
- What are your feelings after eating?
- What are your favorite foods and why?
- What did you learn about food during your childhood?
- Write down your perfect day of healthy eating.
- Write down your goals for weight management and your life.
- How has your perception of food changed in the last week, month, or year?
- What bad habits and food relationships do you need to eliminate from your life?
- What are your favorite hobbies or pastimes you could do instead of eating?
- Dear body, I want to embark on mindful eating because...
- I love myself because...

Journaling provides inspiration for future success. It can help you understand yourself better and allow you to accept yourself for who you are while building productive habits. It enables you to have a positive image to work towards and provides motivation for healthy eating.

Make Small Changes

Coping with your emotions requires constant practice just like mindful eating does. It is not an easy process and you need to be kind to yourself along the way. Sometimes, you go full force into a new activity but it becomes unsustainable in the long-term because the change is too big. It is much better to start with small changes and build up to a life of healthy habits. This strategy ensures you master one concept before moving to another one. The ideas below are small changes you can make to help you and you can add some of your own ideas as you see fit.

A Month of Mindful Eating

Commit to being aware of your emotions for one month. As soon as you start to think about food, write down how you are feeling before you eat and after you have eaten. Make notes about your emotions, when and where you experience them, and why. Write down what you want to eat and what you decided to eat. Do this every time you are prompted to eat.

Choose an Emotion

Check your notes from the month, and identify the emotion that comes up most frequently. You only need to choose one emotion. The others will have a turn at a later stage. For this exercise, let's use stress as the main emotion in the notes.

Find Coping Strategies

Determine how you can deal with this emotion in a healthy way. For example, you could deal with stress through meditation, exercise, or reading instead of eating.

Focus on the Trigger

Whenever you feel the urge to eat, identify the predominant emotion at that time. This emotion is triggering your eating, so if you identify it as stress (for example), then move on to the next step.

Use the New Technique

After identifying the trigger as the reason you want to eat, it is time to take action. Bring your list of coping strategies for this emotion into play, even if it is just for a short while. For example, you could do the relaxation meditation, go for a brisk five-minute walk, or read a couple of pages from your favorite book. Allow the new technique to take the place of eating until the urge to eat passes.

Get Support

Involve your family and friends in your emotional and weight loss journey. It helps to find an accountability partner with whom you can talk to daily about how you fared with the emotion you are treating. Many times, an accountability partner can help you through your emotion, if you call upon them when you struggle to practice the coping strategy. They can talk to you for a few minutes or go on a walk with you to help distract you from your emotional craving.

Repeat

Once you have one emotion under control (about a month later), repeat the process with the next most prevalent emotion on your list. Remain patient, you can succeed.

Take Five

Mindless eating becomes an automatic event, but you can stop it if you press pause for a few moments. Stop in your tracks whenever a craving hits or you feel like eating. While you are paying attention to yourself, you can consider why you have a craving and decide to take a different course of action. The most important thing is to take five minutes, that is all.

Ask yourself whether you can wait to eat for five minutes. If that seems like too big a challenge, then wait for one minute, and another minute, and another, until you reach five minutes. Be patient with yourself, and continuously request yourself to wait. It's not that you won't eat, you just need some time to think before you eat.

Check-in with your emotions and hunger while you take five. Determine your prevailing emotions, measure your hunger on the relevant scale, and try to find a different way to deal with the craving. Write down these emotions and other information, especially if you do decide to eat something, so that you can understand your decision later on.

Do Something Else

What would you do if you cannot eat right now? Try to name at least five things you could do instead of eating and write them down in your journal. The easiest way to overcome mindless eating is to do something else when you want to eat. Here are several things you could do when a craving hits.

Visualize

Your imagination is a powerful tool. Use it to entertain yourself and distract you from food cravings.

- Visualize yourself full of energy.
- Imagine yourself at your dream weight.
- Paint a picture of bliss.
- Visualize a healthy meal.
- Think about your dreams for the future.

Get Moving

When you move, you release the same feel-good hormones as when you are eating. Start moving and feeling good without the guilt of food.

- Take a walk around the block.
- Dance.
- Play an instrument.
- Wash your car.
- Do some gardening.
- Fit new clothes.

Spend Time with Others

Socialization is an excellent way to bust cravings. It gives you time to think of something else than food.

- Call a friend.
- Read a book to children.
- Volunteer at a local charity.
- Play a board game.
- Attend an event.

Look After Yourself

Self-love is essential if you want to move forward on your weight management journey. Appreciate your body and who you are by taking care of it properly.

- Go for a massage.
- Thank yourself for your hard work.
- Take a nap.
- Go for a manicure and pedicure.
- Buy flowers for yourself.

Express Yourself

Don't bottle up your emotions, instead, let them out. When you release emotions, you set yourself free.

- Write down your top ten reasons to exercise.
- Journal.
- Scream.
- Write a thank you note to someone.
- Pray.

Declutter Your Life

An organized life leads to an organized mind. Start to sort out the clutter around you, and it will have a positive mental effect.

- Fold the laundry.
- Wash the dishes.
- Write down a to-do list.
- Plan your vacation.
- Create a meal plan.
- Clear a junk drawer.
- Complete an unfinished project.
- List your priorities and goals.

Choose your favorite options from the lists above. Make a shortlist with your top five to ten ideas and carry it with you wherever you go. Pull out your list as soon as you feel a craving, and put your distraction tactics to the test.

Ideas for Specific Emotions

All these activities may seem a little overwhelming and abstract at first. It helps to have ideas for when you experience specific emotions so that you have a quick strategy to deal with your cravings. Here are some ideas.

Stress

Start exercising to get your blood pumping. Break fitness down into a set number of squats, push ups, burpees, or star jumps at a time. Try jogging, cycling, or swimming if you want to put distance between yourself and the stressful event. Yoga or pilates provides a challenge and improves awareness, as it requires your full concentration. Do a meditation exercise, go for a neck and shoulder massage, breathe deeply, and drink lots of water.

Celebrations

When you achieve something amazing you want to celebrate, and you should, but don't turn to food. Find another reward. Treat yourself to a new outfit or hobby equipment. Feed your emotion with an adrenaline-filled activity, like rock climbing or mountain biking. Take a bubble bath, have sex, or go for a beauty treatment.

Seeking Comfort (Loneliness, Sadness, and Depression)

After a long day or difficult event, there is nothing better than a bowl of your favorite comfort food. Now, is the time to change this habit, and find other ways of getting comfort. Ask a friend to come over for a chat, give someone a hug, and watch a feel-good movie. Snuggle up in your favorite blanket, or play with your pets. Meditate or do yoga. Have a cup of tea. Find solace in nature and watch a sunset. A candle-lit bubble bath with soft background music does a world of good.

Boredom

Mindless eating occurs when you are bored, so it is time to ditch this feeling. Make a list of things you have been putting off and want to get done. Choose one item off this list each time you feel bored, and complete this task when you identify boredom. Clean your room, sort out your closet, wash the car, or do some filing. Change rooms and spend some time reading, painting, or journaling. Listen to music, call a friend, or get some exercise.

Socialization

Eating and socializing are frequent partners, so you need to get your social circle to help you out with this one. Choose something else to do than eat. You could play a team sport, go for a hike or bike ride, or go dancing. Consider going bowling, attending a paint night, or watching a movie. Walking with friends during your lunch hour is helpful, and challenge each other to attend charity fun runs.

Towards a Positive Future

Mindfulness assists you to cope with problems in an effective and healthy manner. Using the strategies in this chapter, you will reduce negative thoughts while increasing your self-confidence. Mindfulness will help you to gain control over your life, decrease overwhelming feelings, and allow you to identify eating triggers. Use these coping mechanisms frequently and as a collaborative tool with mindful eating.

Chapter 8: Mindfulness and Eating Disorders

Eating disorders refer to an array of psychological conditions resulting in the development of unhealthy eating habits. It could start as a food obsession, food aversion, issues with body weight and shape. Many people hide their eating disorders because they fear judgment by others, but leaving these disorders untreated can lead to detrimental health and even death in extreme cases. Consult a doctor if you think you have an eating disorder so that they can help you get your health back on track.

Mindfulness is a popular part of treatments for eating disorders. It is useful to help you focus on the positive things and assists in separating your psychological state from your eating habits. Both binge eaters and emotional eaters benefit from mindful eating practices.

Binge Eating

Binge eating is a prevalent eating disorder and one that you might not realize you have. A binge refers to a period of time in which you consume a lot of food in an attempt to escape your emotions. About 70% of obese individuals engage in binge eating, but mindful eating can decrease binge eating by more than 50% (Bjarnadottir, 2019). Binge eating is different from overeating since binge eating occurs even when a person isn't hungry at all. Soon after a binge, you will feel guilty or ashamed about your actions.

Symptoms

There are various signs of being a binge eater. You might sneak snacks, sometimes a whole grocery run full, into your room, eat them in secret, and then hide the evidence. Another example is buying a cake for friends but finishing it alone, which is followed by guilt. You might find yourself ordering three meals and a milkshake from a fast food restaurant and eating everything, resulting in feelings of uncomfortable fullness. This is different to occasional overeating, which could be seen as mindlessly eating a large popcorn during a movie.

Other symptoms of binge eating include:

- Eating until you feel uncomfortably full
- Eating alone to avoid embarrassment
- Eating very quickly
- Eating without hunger cues
- Experiencing sadness, loneliness, guilt, and disgust

If you find yourself eating vast amounts of food in a short time and feel that this behavior is out of control, then you need to consider your situation carefully. Binge eaters need instant gratification and, although you might consume food so quickly it becomes mindless, you need the food to feel better about yourself, even if it is for a very short time. You may have a binge eating disorder if you binge at least once weekly for longer than three months.

Reasons for Binge Eating

There are many reasons why a person may become a binge eater. Some reasons are based on emotional issues while others have their roots in family matters. Whatever the reason for your binge eating, you need to address the situation immediately to get your health back.

Genes

Binge eating can become a family affair, as it could be part of your genetics. If a parent or grandparent was a binge eater, then you may have the same binge eating gene, which increases your chances of falling victim to this eating disorder. The genes responsible for binge eating cues affect networks in your brain that normally control mood and appetite. Having a binge eating gene does not mean that you will become a binge eater—this disorder has to be triggered by something else.

Copycat Eating

Your family and upbringing affect your eating habits. Adults set an example for children, so your binge eating may have been something you learned from family members. Be very careful if you have children or other individuals looking up to you; you don't want to influence their eating habits negatively. Binge eating must be treated, but if you are struggling, then do not binge in front of impressionable individuals.

Extreme Dieting

Diets place restrictions on your food choices and consumption, which later leads to binge eating. When following a diet, you may have to skip meals, eat too little, or really just need a cheat day. Instead of treating yourself, you could find yourself binge eating everything not allowed on your diet plan. Of course, this results in guilty feelings and you may find yourself eating even more.

Depression

A link between depression and binge eating does exist, but the exact cause-and-effect is still murky. Researchers are trying to understand whether guilt and shame from binge eating cause depression, or whether it is the other way round. Regardless, approximately half of binge eaters also have depression, so consider it a warning sign if both are present in your life.

Stress and Anxiety

Traumatic or stressful events can lead a person to overeat. Usually, this is a short-term occurrence, and the person returns to healthy eating habits once the stress is removed. You might have experienced overeating before tests or after losing a friend. This relates closely to emotional eating. If this situation is left untreated or if you let it get out of control, you may find that you frequently binge at the smallest sign of stress.

Low Self-Esteem

When you are unhappy about your body, you feel bad about yourself, which leads to low self-esteem. This could be the result of your own beliefs or something that someone else had said. Browsing through social media and magazines doesn't help the situation either, because the media portrays bodies differently from what they look like in reality. Low self-esteem may cause binge eating and extreme guilt resulting in a downwards spiral.

Binge eating remains a health risk and has many complications. If you binge, you may experience anxiety, depression, and other psychological problems. You also increase your risk of developing diabetes, hypertension, and heart disease, which makes you susceptible to stroke and organ damage.

Mindful Eating to Overcome Binge Eating Disorder

Binge eating results in negative emotions after rapid, excessive eating. In contrast, mindful eating focuses on the eating experience and moderation. Mindfulness is an ideal treatment for binge eating. It allows you to see yourself objectively while remaining aware of the current moment. Mindfulness breaks down the protective barriers you set up with binge eating and enables you to see recovery in a healthy manner. Mindful eating allows you to see food as a nutritional tool rather than as a coping mechanism. In turn, you can deal with your binge eating triggers in an effective manner.

Mindfulness can help you to overcome binge eating by reducing negative thoughts and enables you to build your confidence through proper eating. If you are a binge eater or feel a binge eating episode coming on, then you could follow the next steps to help you become a healthy, mindful eater.

Recognize Your Hunger

Use the hunger scale frequently during the day to help you establish if how hungry you are at that moment. Eat something as soon as you rate your hunger as a three or four. Avoid reaching the one or two-level, because you will be so hungry by that time that you will be more likely to overeat, which could result in binging. Evaluate your hunger after 15 to 20 minutes of eating, and stop when you reach a level six or seven. If you still feel hungry, then allow 15 minutes to pass before you eat something else. You might find you now feel full and won't fall prey to binging.

Remove Binge-Worthy Foods

You probably have a list of favorite foods for binging. It could be chocolate, cake, chips, a fast food meal, ice cream, or something else. Clear your house of all these foods so that you do not become tempted through cravings.

Concentrate on Your Food

Use as many mindfulness techniques while eating as possible. Switch off devices and screens to avoid becoming distracted, sit at the table to eat, and do not try to multitask while eating.

Use a Food Journal

Write down all the foods you eat and how you feel when eating. Study your food journal for triggers. It also helps you identify if you really ate too much or whether this is a figment of your imagination.

Replace Boredom With Activity

Boredom frequently leads to binge eating, especially if you are alone and start to feel sad or depressed. Find activities to do in your spare time instead of lying around at home. Being productive makes it easier to remain positive and doesn't leave time for binge eating.

Binge eating is a serious food disorder that can point to underlying emotional or psychological issues. Once you deal with these problems you can overcome binge eating. Mindful eating is the ideal lifestyle change if you struggle from binge eating because you can still enjoy your favorite foods albeit in a more responsible way.

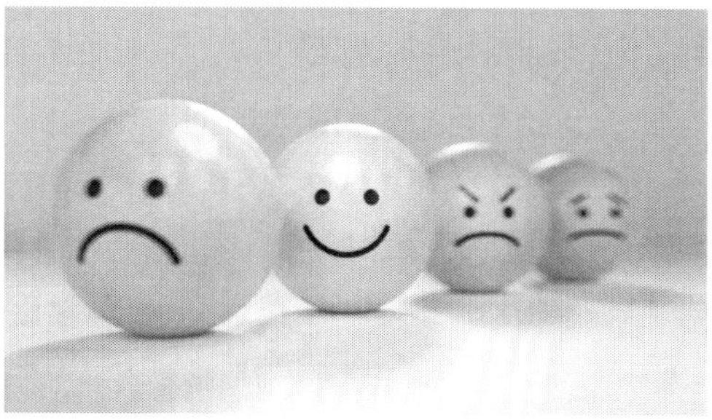

Emotional Eating

Emotional eating occurs when you decide to cope with your emotions by eating. Some people refer to this situation as, "eating their emotions" because they are not hungry physically but they seek comfort from food. This "comfort" actually comes from the release of feel-good hormones in the biological loop.

Symptoms of Emotional Eating

You probably have a good idea if you are an emotional eater because you know you reach for food when your emotions ride a rollercoaster. You may eat when you are stressed, sad, anxious, bored, happy, angry, or other emotions. You eat in the hope of feeling better, as you believe it will calm you down or make you happier. Emotional eaters use food as a reward for doing something good, or as a reward for getting through a tough situation. You may eat even if you are not hungry and you could be eating after you reach satiation. Food might be a safe haven for you, a friend who supports you when you need emotional help.

Causes of Emotional Eating

Emotional eating doesn't just happen. There is some precursor that causes you to grab food to deal with your emotions. At its core, it is an emotion that triggers this compulsive behavior, but understanding what causes this emotion will help shed light on your choices.

Childhood Habits

Most of your habits in adulthood come from what you were taught as a child. Your parents might have rewarded you for a good school term by taking you for ice cream, gave you a candy bar after falling, or purchased takeaways for the family if a parent had a busy day. All of these actions were done with good intentions, but they taught you that eating when emotional is okay. Now, you repeat the same actions in your adult life.

Stress

Stress can make you more hungry resulting in overeating. Chronic stress generates a hormone called cortisol, which produces cravings for sweet, salty, and fried foods. All of these foods allow for a quick release of feel-good hormones and provide energy. If you cannot control your stress, then you will be at risk for emotional eating.

Numbing Emotions

Emotional eating is an avoidance behavior. When you experience unwanted emotions, you may decide to eat something, rather than face your emotional instability. Ignoring your emotions is not the solution to your problems. You need to address the real situation to set yourself free from emotional eating.

Feeling Empty

Sometimes, you feel as if you have a void in your life. This could be due to boredom or feeling empty. If you experience this emptiness, then you might decide to fill it with food. Eating is a distraction when you feel you have no purpose or are uncertain about how to achieve satisfaction.

Social Influences

Social settings easily cause overeating and emotional eating. You may become nervous or stressed in social circles and start to eat as a coping mechanism. The excitement and happiness of spending time with others can elicit great joy too, which may lead to celebratory eating.

It is always a good idea to determine the cause(s) of your emotional eating. It helps you to address the real problem, and you can identify emotional triggers. Identifying the cause might not happen overnight, and it could be quite complex, but the investigation will increase your mindfulness.

Emotional Eating Cycle

Food can be used as a reward or a pick-me-up on occasion. It is not a problem if you do it this way, but you cannot let it become a compulsive behavior. If eating becomes your primary coping mechanism for emotional circumstances, then you may soon face the perpetual emotional eating cycle.

There are four steps in the cycle:

- You become upset about something.
- You have an overwhelming craving for food.
- You overeat, even though you know better.
- You feel ashamed and guilty.

This cycle continues on and on. You can start at any point in this cycle and will soon realize that you circle on to the other steps. It is very difficult to get out of this cycle, and you will beat yourself up because it feels like you are failing. The only way to escape this vicious cycle is to learn better ways to cope with your emotions. Mindfulness is one strategy to help you overcome emotional instability.

Difference Between Emotional Hunger and Physical Hunger

A big problem with emotional eating is that people do not recognize it as emotions, but rather assume it is hunger. Separating emotions from hunger is essential if you want to overcome emotional eating. The differences between these concepts may seem a bit vague in your daily life, but mindful eaters become more aware, and this will help you identify what you are really experiencing.

Here is a comparison.

- Emotional hunger starts quickly while physical hunger builds gradually.
- Emotional hunger presents as thoughts of eating whereas physical hunger manifests within your stomach.
- Emotional hunger appears as sharp, incessant cravings while physical hunger generates growling sounds that occur off-an-on.
- Emotional hunger is satisfied by certain foods, textures, or tastes, while physical hunger is satisfied by any food, even ones you do not prefer.
- Emotional eating is challenging to satisfy, and most people eat too much, but physical hunger only requires a regular portion of food to feel satisfied.
- Emotional eating may result in feelings of shame, regret, and guilt after eating, whereas physical hunger doesn't cause negative feelings.

Become Mindful of Your Emotions

Mindfulness can help you sort through your emotions. It allows you to become aware of what you are feeling without judgment and to embrace these emotions. Here is a technique for emotional mindfulness:

- Take a few deep breaths.
- Tell yourself: "It is okay to feel (insert emotion)."

- Name the emotion and welcome it into your being, even if it has negative qualities.
- Remain neutral in your attitude towards the emotions, but have a sense of curiosity and kindness.
- Ask the emotion what it wants from you and truly listen to the requests from your inner being.
- Thank the emotion for sharing these insights, and tell it you will work on improving the situation.
- Take a few deep breaths and then continue with your next activities.

This quick exercise enables you to tune into your body's needs. It allows your body to find peace and ensures it that you will protect it in other ways, rather than creating a defense through food. You can also use this process as writing prompts for your food journal.

Feeding Your Feelings

Becoming a mindful eater is an excellent choice if you struggle with emotional eating. There are so many mindful eating activities and tools that can help you determine whether you experience physical or emotional hunger, and these tools can help you beat your emotional cravings. Overcoming emotional eating is a challenge, but you can do it with determination and grit.

As you start out on mindful eating, you have to realize that you won't always be able to say no to emotional eating. There will be times when you find yourself searching for food because nothing else brings you satisfaction. When this happens, you should keep in mind three principles. These three principles will help you to remain a mindful eater during emotional eating episodes.

1. Accept that emotional eating is a choice you make to help you cope with a situation. Coping is not a failure, so emotional eating cannot be a failure either, and no reason exists to feel guilty.
2. Follow the mindful eating principles when you eat emotionally. This means you have to eat with awareness, remain in the moment, sit at the table, avoid other distractions, and so on. The eating period should have an identifiable start and finish times to avoid mindless eating.
3. Emotional eating does not require overeating. Stop eating when your hunger level is at a five or six on the hunger scale.

Emotional eating can help you to overcome a current situation if you remain mindful throughout the process. Mindful eating should become a ritual that you can apply regardless of your circumstances because it focuses on awareness. Use your mindful eating techniques to slow down your snowballing emotions, so that you eat sensibly and without feelings of shame or guilt.

Conquer Emotional Eating

Deciding to change from an emotional eater to a mindful eater is a big step. You should be proud of yourself for wanting to cope with your emotions better and in healthier ways. Finding alternative coping strategies is important if you want to replace emotional eating once and for all. Whenever you feel a bout of emotional eating coming on, take a moment to identify the underlying emotion. Once you name the motion, you can use a suitable technique to cope. If you feel lonely or depressed, then doing something to lift your spirits like reminiscing about a good time with friends, paging through a photo album, or playing with your pets. Deal with anxiety and stress by transferring your nervous energy through dancing, mediation, yoga, or clenching a stress ball. Exhaustion can be overcome by taking a hot shower or bath, using aromatherapy and essential oils, drinking a cup of tea, and taking a nap.

Beat Eating Disorders

Any change in eating habits is difficult, even more so when the habit is part of your very existence and a means of coping. Eating disorders have no place in your life, so take back control of your eating and beat binge and emotional eating. Keep a positive attitude, immerse yourself in other activities, and congratulate yourself for the small victories. You have all the power within you to transform your life, and mindfulness can help you manifest this strength to manage your eating behaviors.

Chapter 9: Mindful Eating and Weight Loss

Weight loss is a hot topic in most conversations. Everywhere you go, you will hear people talking about their weight and how they are attempting to lose a few pounds for this reason or that event. Society constantly pushes the idea of the "perfect" size, but it is unrealistic and only leads to unhealthy eating behaviors.

Think about yourself and your close social circle for a moment. Identify some destructive weight loss behaviors they exhibit. Some people skip meals, decide to fast, or only eat cauliflower and chicken for a month. There are hundreds of fad diets and so-called "quick fixes" that promise weight loss in the blink of an eye. This is unrealistic and unhealthy.

You have to feed your body properly if you want to be healthy. Yes, you might be able to cut down on portion sizes, your sugar, and caffeine consumption, and limit your snacking. All of these things are good, but you can do all of these things in moderation and without restriction through mindful eating. Mindful eating works because it changes your cognitive behavior and lifestyle rather than saying what you can and cannot eat.

Mindful Eating Versus Dieting

How many diets have you been on where you lost the weight and kept it off?

Very few people manage to use short-term diets for long-term weight loss. About 85% of individuals who lose weight by dieting will regain the weight lost (plus a few extra pounds) mere years after their efforts. In contrast, studies using mindful eating found that obese individuals lost weight at a healthy rate and did not regain any weight in subsequent months. Most participants were able to maintain their weight or lost a few more pounds (Bjarnadottir, 2019). Mindful eating is much better than dieting because it changes your approach and behavior towards food while reducing eating-related stress. Mindful eating works since it improves your relationship with food rather than restricting it.

Diets believe that weight loss is possible through willpower alone. You have to use self-discipline to stick to a limited list of foods, ignore your cravings entirely, and only eat at certain times, which will allow you to lose weight. This is wishful thinking. You may be able to cope with the diet mentality for a few days or weeks, but at some time you are going to be emotional, have a craving, or need the energy to continue with your day. You wouldn't deny food to a five-year-old child who says they are physically hungry, yet diets expect you to deny food to yourself, even when you experience real physical hunger.

The problem with diets is that they set high expectations, give you a list of do's and don'ts, but then leave you hanging. Diets label food as food or bad, which causes you to believe that choosing the wrong food makes you a "bad" person. There is no further support to help you through days when your diet is challenging. They don't teach you to cope with your cravings or how to make healthy eating a long-term habit.

Mindful eating is the total opposite of a diet. It is a loose concept focused on eating with awareness. You can eat whatever you want whenever you want as long as you remain mindful of the experience and eat in response to your physical cues. Mindful eating encourages you to listen to what your body needs and respond accordingly. By focusing on internal messages, you increase your awareness and you manage to eat just what you need to satisfy yourself. You allow your body to tell you when it is full, and you have tools like the hunger scale to help you understand these prompts. Mindful eating can help you to lose weight and see food for what it is, a nourishing resource.

Losing weight successfully is an elusive activity. Diets are challenging, especially when you consider how many there are and the variety of their rules. It is tough to decide on the best diet for your body and health concerns. The best diet seems to be the one the media currently advertises, and that can change tomorrow. Some weight loss programs focus on goal setting, like saying you should lose ten pounds in six weeks while others take a behavioral approach and require that you make small adjustments to your eating on a daily basis. Diets may emphasize eating a set number of calories, and require frequent exercise, but both these requirements start to seem like a punishment after a while.

Mindful eating is a bridge between different diets. It places the control in your hands since you know yourself best. It encourages awareness of calories, eating more healthier foods while having smaller portions of special treats, and uses activity including exercise as a way to cope with your cravings and emotions. By concentrating on the journey from mindless eating to mindful eating, you start to realize that the beliefs of diets do have a purpose, but you apply them in a healthier way that is suitable to your personal tastes.

Weight Loss Versus Well-Being

When you decide to lose weight intentionally, you are forcing your body and mind to change their internal processes. This process is called adaptive thermogenesis and alters your psychology, physiology, and biology. Your body is used to maintaining a body fat level based on your nervous system, but you are pushing this storage system to change with intentional weight loss. This sudden change in diet is not something your body takes to kindly, which means it will easily reverse the process if you slip up with your diet.

The changes described above are metabolic in nature, but your body has to adapt biologically too. Your body will resist these immediate changes by altering its chemical balance. For example, restricting your food may cause increased cravings and simultaneously decrease leptin, which is the hormone responsible for feelings of fullness. Additionally, restrictive diets result in distractibility, irritability, and intense emotional responses, especially binge eating and consuming food when not hungry.

The other problem with restrictive diets is that it relies on external information. You learn to eat a set list of foods at certain times, and you have to follow rules set by someone that does not know what your body is experiencing. All of these factors are external to your body. Through this process, you start to distrust the cues from your own body and no longer realize what it is trying to say. You need to relearn how to be self-efficient and trust yourself, which will help to improve your self-esteem.

The best way to get to know yourself is through mindfulness. Mindfulness takes the focus away from weight loss and directs your attention to wellbeing at both a physical and psychological level. It teaches you to look internally for cues about food and to seek new ways to satisfy your real carings. Even if you do not lose weight with mindful eating, your general well-being improves. This leads to general health improvements because you no longer consume less healthy foods in large amounts and you don't overeat. You may find that you have lower cholesterol and blood glucose levels, shorter bouts of depression, fewer food cravings, and a generally positive outlook. These are just some of the benefits you get from focusing on wellbeing rather than on weight loss.

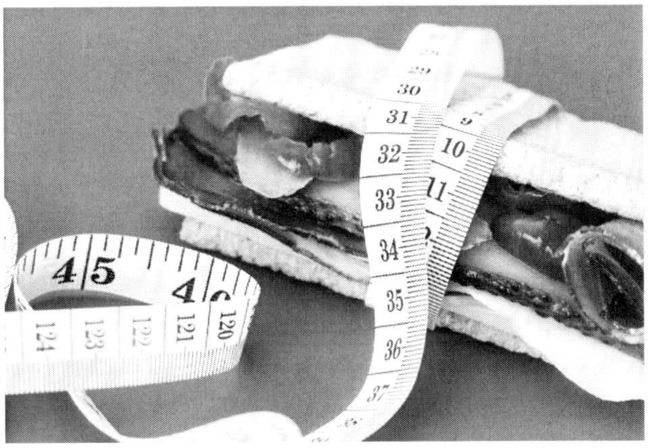

Overeating Triggers

Weight loss with mindfulness is possible, but you need to make changes at the foundation. Being aware of your current situation is one of the best ways to turn from mindless into mindful. It allows you to identify eating triggers, which lead to overeating. At its core, mindless eating resulting in weight gain is due to overeating. Once you identify your overeating triggers, you can limit your exposure to these elements, and start to regain mindful control.

There are three main triggers you should be aware of for mindless overeating.

Distraction

Being distracted is a major factor in overeating. You might not realize how much you eat while you are watching TV, busy with work, or browsing social media. Even general dinnertime conversation can distract you from your food. You need to identify any distractions when eating so that you can address them now. Write down a list of these distractions in a food journal. If you don't enjoy writing, then give yourself a visual cue to distractions by using sticky notes. Place a sticky note on anything that could be a distraction while eating—for example, your cellphone, a wall calendar, an unfinished painting, etc. When you do sit down for a meal, position yourself away from these distractions so that your full attention is on your food.

Emotions

Your emotional state will affect your weight loss efforts. Different emotions affect the hormonal balance in your body even if you are eating only what you should in limited amounts, the hormones in your body could prevent weight loss because the hormones are a defense mechanism. You need to deal with your emotions first, and your weight loss will follow. Go over the section on emotional eating in the previous chapter to help you with this trigger.

Environment

The space you are in at any time of the day could have external cues that entice you to eat. You could be sitting in the car without a morsel of food, look up and see a billboard advertising a bar of chocolate, and end up stopping at the store to buy one. While watching TV and browsing social media you see posts about food and eating. In your own home, you may be confronted with food, even from something harmless such as a photo of a social gathering at a restaurant. Identify these triggers to eat and make a plan on how you will handle them in the future.

Practical Mindful Eating Tips for Weight Loss

You already learned various mindfulness techniques that you can apply to your life. If your plan is to lose weight, then you should definitely go for it, but do not consider it as a punishment. Start to become fully aware of your decision, and embrace the journey to a healthier slimmer you.

Techniques to Reduce Overeating

A huge part of overeating is eating fast and not getting enough to satisfy your cravings. Here are three techniques to take back control of your eating habits. They will help you to become more aware and give your body enough time to send fullness cues which means you stop eating sooner.

Eat In the Dark

A large part of awareness during eating comes from visual cues. You can see how much food you have on your plate, the type of foods, and the colors. Take away your sense of sight to enhance the rest of your senses. You can eat an entire meal in the dark at night, close your eyes for a few bites, or use a blindfold. When you cannot see what is on your plate, you have to rely on your taste buds to give you information. You are less tempted to eat everything because you have to eat slower, which allows you to realize satiation cues. Eating in the dark could lead to much smaller portion sizes, and you can use this as an indicator for future portions.

Switch It Up

You eat faster and more when you have the right utensils. Changing your utensils entirely, as seen in Chapter Six, can help you to eat slower and be more aware of your eating. Do this frequently if you are overeating and want to lose weight.

A Taste Bud Curveball

The first bite of food always tastes amazing, but subsequent bites lose this effect. This leads to eating more because you seek the same experience you had with the first bite. Your taste buds start to recognize the taste and get used to it, so eating the rest is less appealing, yet you continue to eat in search of satisfaction. If you experience this, take a bite of a different food that has another temperature, texture, or flavor. Wait a few seconds, then return to the first food and take another bite. Determine if it tastes different and now satisfies you. If it doesn't, then accept that you won't have the same experience as the first bite and walk away from this food item.

Interview With Yourself

Mindfulness requires a keen interest in yourself and the communication given by your body. When you are trying to lose weight, you are constantly faced with wanting to eat and need to learn your body's cues to understand what it really wants. This situation takes time and practice. One way to help you build a sense of hunger knowledge is to have an interview with yourself whenever you feel the urge to eat. You can also use this strategy if you already put food into your mouth mindlessly, as it will help understand what drove you to this action.

The main question you want to answer is why you are eating. You need to investigate whether you are hungry. This is very difficult to know because the chances of experiencing real physical hunger are very slim since it isn't something you are exposed to frequently. There are three questions that can help you understand your hunger and whether you should be eating.

1. Do I Need To Eat?

If you really need to eat, then you will experience physical hunger cues. You either need energy through calories, macronutrients from proteins, fats, and carbohydrates, micronutrients like vitamins and minerals, or a combination of these. When you need to eat, you could have physical cues such as tiredness, a rumbling stomach, or dizziness. These signals should alert you to the fact that eating cannot be put off any longer.

2. Do I Want To Eat?

If you simply want to eat, it is usually because you are craving something that tastes good. Your craving could be for something that is not nutritious and loaded with salt, sugar, and fat. An enjoyable or favorite flavor and texture could be right at the top of the list. You will have a sudden desire to eat these foods, so wait a few minutes for the craving to pass. If you do give in to temptation, then take a very small portion and consume it mindfully.

3. Do I Feel Like I Should Eat?

There are some situations where you feel that you should be eating, but you may not be hungry at all. Question whether your current environment or external cues are the reason behind eating in this case. You do not need to conform to social norms, so rather turn to a different activity or measure your hunger on the appropriate scale before eating unnecessarily.

Some Other Ideas

Here are some more ideas and tips to help you with your weight loss efforts. All of these ideas promote mindfulness.

Get Enough Sleep

Sleeping too little makes you hungrier and you are more likely to eat when you wake up. Sleep at least eight hours per night. Practice mindfulness before you go to bed to help you focus on sleeping. Switch off all digital devices, do relaxation exercises or meditation, and be grateful as you lay down to sleep. When you do wake up the next morning, take a moment to be thankful for the new day, and evaluate your hunger using the hunger scale before deciding to grab a snack for mindless munching.

Meal Plan

Planning your meals is a good way to improve your mindfulness. It gives some structure to your food choices and helps you to know what you are going to eat. If you have an idea of what you can eat on a specific day, you will eat smaller portions and be less prone to snacking because you don't have to wonder about what you are going to eat. Use your meal plan to write a grocery list, and only purchase the food items on your list in reasonable amounts. Prepare the food once you get home by cutting up vegetables, marinating meat, and so on. By preparing your food in advance and portioning it properly, you become less tempted to grab something quickly or out of convenience. Pre-portioning also helps you to eat less, and you can always use the two-plate approach if you think you are still overeating.

Eat More Plant-Based Foods

Vegetables have fewer calories, so bulk up on them if you feel you need to eat a bit more. A cup of cucumber has almost no calories compared to several hundred in a cup of pasta. You should avoid overeating at all times. If you eat more vegetables, you can repeat the hunger measurement frequently during your meal and stop eating sooner, which means you are consuming fewer calories but still feel full.

Reward Yourself

You are working hard at being healthier and eating well. Reward yourself occasionally for your efforts by eating something you really love. Buy or prepare it as a much smaller portion and only serve yourself half of what you think you could eat. Enjoy this item while keeping all your mindful eating techniques in place. Stop eating when you feel just a bit full to avoid overeating and try some of the utensil swapping techniques to heighten the experience.

Mindful Eating During Holidays

The holidays and any other celebratory event are a challenge if you are trying to lose weight. You might be one of those people who diet in advance and loses a few pounds so that you can eat more during the holidays. This situation only leads to overeating and feeling ill afterward. It's also very difficult to continue with a diet if you stopped it during the holidays. Mindful eating makes the holidays much easier—it is not a diet, so it is easier to maintain as long as you remain mindful.

Social Strategy

You know the hallmarks of your holidays and what to expect. If your family and friends usually have food at get-togethers, then offer to take a snack platter or dish. You can fill the dish with wholesome, healthy choices, such as carrot and celery sticks, cherry tomatoes, and sliced fruit. Taking a healthy snack platter to an event ensures that you have a healthier alternative if you do get the munchies.

Holidays are full of social distractions, so place yourself as far away from the food and alcoholic beverages as possible. Do not be tempted to talk to the hosts in the kitchen or dining room, and do not get caught up in conversation near a food table. If you do want to talk to someone, then ask them if they could have a walk around the party with you. It will give you some time to move and you purposefully move away from any tempting foods.

Increased Awareness

Keep all your mindful eating strategies in mind beforehand while you attend an event. Evaluate your hunger level, if you feel cravings setting in, and only eat if it is physical hunger. Savor every bite by being aware of the smells, tastes, textures, and colors of the food. It can be challenging to eat mindfully when you are around many people, so it might be easiest to find a quiet area in the garden to eat in peace. If you are having a sit-down meal, then use the two-plate approach, or decide to eat only half of what is on your plate, and reevaluate your hunger before you eat the rest. Be thankful for each item on your plate and put down your utensils between bites which ensures you experience your food fully.

A New You

A healthy body weight is a noble cause because it shows you care about your health and want to improve yourself. Mindful eating allows you to realize this goal by strengthening the connection between mind and body. By focusing more on wellbeing, you empower yourself to make better decisions and start to lose weight through proactive activities. Weight loss can be a slow process but have hope—you will succeed, build a positive self-image, and have a better relationship with eating in the process.

Chapter 10: FAQ

Everything you need to know about mindful eating is in this book. If you are still wondering about some things, then you may find the information below to be useful.

What is Mindful Eating?

Mindful eating forms part of the concept of mindfulness. It means to stay in the moment. With mindful eating, you use various techniques to enhance your awareness of your relationship with food. In turn, this allows you to eat sensibly and in a controlled manner that is beneficial for your health.

Is Mindful Eating a Diet?

No, mindful eating is a practice to increase your awareness of the eating process. It is not a diet, which restricts food or calories. Mindful eating does encourage you to be calorie conscious, consider your food options carefully and eat slower. In the process, mindful eating results in eating healthier and less because you feel full sooner which has similar effects to a diet.

Who Can Become a Mindful Eater?

Mindful eating is suitable for everyone, regardless of age, gender, and other demographic factors. You can teach your children and other family members to become mindful eaters. It is suitable if you have health problems like diabetes and high blood pressure because it generates healthy eating behavior that frequently decreases the extent of your diagnosis. As with any change in your lifestyle, it is advisable to consult a healthcare practitioner before you start practicing mindful eating.

How is Mindful Eating Different From Intuitive Eating?

The concept of mindful eating refers to being aware of what and how you eat. Intuitive eating includes mindfulness, but it is a model with ten principles and three elements. Intuitive eating has more rigid guidelines when compared to mindful eating.

Will Mindful Eating Stop Me From Eating the Foods I Like?

No. You can enjoy any food when you are a mindful eater. The most important thing is to remain aware of the eating process and signals from your body. Mindful eating will help you to determine proper portion size, enhance the sensory experience while eating, and allow you to feel full sooner so you are eating less.

Will Mindful Eating Change My Life?

Mindful eating can change your life as you embark on a journey of sensory stimulation, become one with your body, and have a healthy relationship with food. Mindful eating is part of a large concept called mindfulness. With mindfulness, you are fully present in the current moment and immerse yourself in the experience. Mindful eating will change an aspect of your life while mindfulness will change your whole life.

Can Mindful Eating Cure my Eating Disorder?

Mindful eating can help you overcome eating disorders in a healthy way. It gives you techniques and strategies to understand the underlying causes of your eating disorder and provides tools to help you cope with this problem. Mindful eating is a great way to change your eating habits, but you should always see a doctor about an eating disorder so that they can help you with appropriate treatment.

Can I Lose Weight With Mindful Eating?

Absolutely! Mindful eating practices help you to enjoy food without constant overeating. It teaches you to stay in tune with your body without limiting your choice of or access to food. Have a look at Chapter Nine for more information about weight loss through mindful eating.

What Should I Do if I Forget to Eat Mindfully?

Everyone slips up now and then. Do not punish yourself for this mishap since you are already correcting your behavior by acknowledging mindless eating. Go through the mindful eating activities and exercise in this book to refresh your memory. You can also prepare to eat mindfully with your next meal by printing using the hunger scale, keeping a food journal, and using different utensils. There are so many mindful eating tips that you will soon be back on track.

How Do I Know If I am Eating Mindfully?

Mindful eating is a personal process. If you are doing anything to become more aware of your eating and food, then you are starting to be more mindful. Mindfulness does not happen overnight. You need to practice it daily, even if it is for one meal or a few minutes. The more you use the activities and techniques in this book, the more proficient you will become at mindful eating. The mere fact that you are asking this question already shows that you are thinking about eating differently, which is an indicator of mindfulness. Keep going, you will soon see drastic changes as your mindfulness practices take shape.

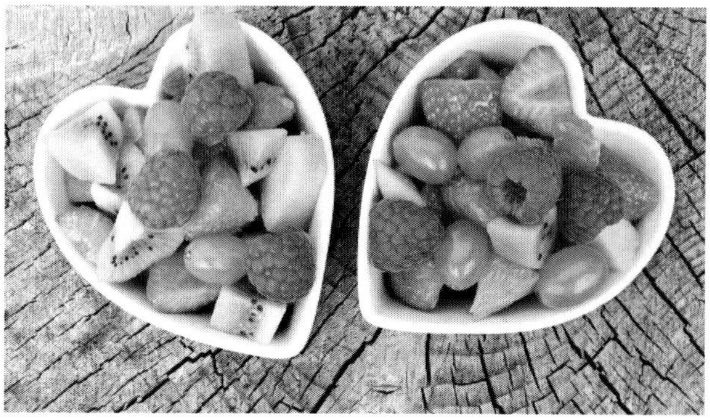

I Am Worried About Eating the Wrong Thing. How Can I Prevent This?

There are no right or wrong things in mindful eating. The belief is that all food is good for you, but some foods have better nutritional content than others. For example, pumpkin is a better choice than fried chicken since pumpkin does not contain all the oils and added ingredients that fried chicken does. Mindful eating wants you to be conscious of the calories and nutritional content in your foods, so if a food is high in calories, then the best option would be to eat a smaller portion of it or only eat it on a special occasion.

Whenever you think a food is "wrong," take some time to research the food, its ingredients, and get a rough idea about the calories. Having this information gives you the power to make a suitable decision. You should always follow the mindful eating guidelines, but even more so with a food that is considered to be less healthy. Mindful eating will enhance your experience of the food and make it more enjoyable. Listen to the cues from your body and stop eating when you feel you are starting to become full. Stay focused and celebrate the small achievements.

How Do I Know If I Should Eat?

Are you hungry or do you think you should be hungry? If you aren't hungry, then you don't need to eat. The best way to determine whether you are hungry is to use the hunger scale to measure your hunger level. Only eat if your hunger measures four or less, meaning you are a bit hungry to ravenous. Be wary of eating because societal norms dictate that you should eat at a certain time or because everyone else is eating.

Where Should I Start With the Mindful Eating Process?

First, you should be proud of yourself for deciding to make this change. Reading this book is a great starting point. It will give you the tools to become a mindful eater. Have a look at Chapter Five to become familiar with the mindful eating principles and the basic tools. You can also use Chapter Six for some mindfulness exercises that will help you to make it a part of your daily life. Small changes are all you need to get started on this process, and you can gradually build up to making mindful eating a full-time practice.

How Should I Deal With Cravings?

Cravings are a symptom of a problem just like a sore throat could signify you are getting a cold. You need to identify what your cravings are trying to tell you. Test your craving to determine whether you have physical or emotional hunger. Use the hunger scale to help you decide if you should eat. Alternatively, deal with emotional hunger by identifying the underlying emotion and do an activity to distract you from your craving. You can find some activity ideas in Chapter Seven.

I Really Love Cooking. Can I Still Cook Like I Did Before?

Yes, you can still cook. You might find that your cooking style and ingredient choice changes when you practice mindfulness. You could switch out traditional cooking oil for a healthier alternative, might fry foods less, and opt for healthier cooking methods like grilling, steaming, or juicing. Preparing and cooking food is part of mindfulness because it gives you an appreciation of the raw ingredients and preparation process. Concentrate on the textures and colors of the raw ingredients and how they change while cooking. All of these small things help to increase your mindfulness, so you should continue to cook.

How Do I Remain A Mindful Eater When Going Out?

Keep your mindful eating principles in mind while eating. Only order a small portion, such as a starter, and use the two-plate approach to help you determine how much you should eat. If you are not going out for a meal, but to watch a movie or socialize, then eat something before you go if you are hungry and measure your hunger level when you get to the event. Only eat something if you are still hungry. You will succeed because you already made the choice to improve your life.

Leave a 1-Click Review!

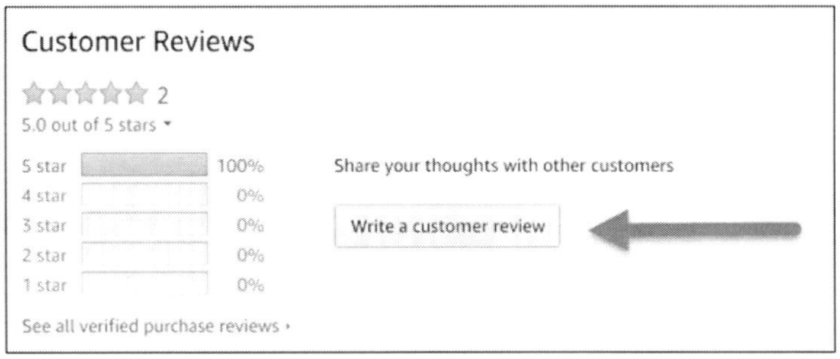

I would be incredibly thankful if you could take just 60 seconds to write a brief review on Amazon, even if it's just a few sentences!

>> Scan with your camera to leave a quick review:

Thank you and I can't wait to see your thoughts.

Conclusion

"When practiced to its fullest, mindful eating turns a simple meal into a spiritual experience, giving us a deep appreciation of all that went into the meal's creation as well as a deep understanding of the relationship between the food on our table, or own health, and our planet's health." - Thich Nhat Hanh, Buddhist monk and peace activist who lives according to mindfulness principles.

How has your life changed since you started the process of becoming a mindful eater?

Visualize your before and after scenarios for a moment, just like you would take before and after photos when on a weight-loss initiative. Create an image titled, "Before Mindful Eating," and another titled "After Mindful Eating." Consider how your life has changed in the process. Your before image might be of yourself and your family eating a whole pizza each while drinking soda and staring blankly at the TV. In your after visualization, you depict your new reality: a family eating together at the table, sharing a single pizza, understanding satiation cues, and talking about the food experience.

Take your visualization one step further. Think about the type of mindful eater you want to be in a year's time. You might see yourself losing weight, being healthier, more energetic, and have a lust for life. Your relationship with food could be even better, you might have planted a few fruits, vegetables, and herbs yourself, and junk food has a very small role in your life. What a great place to be in! Hold onto this vision as you continue to eat mindfully.

Your relationship with food is an important part of your life. It will always be there, so you need to learn how to improve this relationship in a healthy way. Food is an existential piece of our existence. Food is an amazing thing because it comes from the earth, just like you do. You have a connection with the earth through your consumption of food. Every bite of food you take is the sum of nature's efforts. The whole universe—sun, moon, ground, and water—work together to provide amazing produce for you to consume. You should do this with happiness and enjoyment, instead of with feelings of guilt and shame. Once you learn to eat properly through mindful eating, you gain the ability to strengthen your connection to food and the earth.

Mindful eating is the perfect healthy lifestyle choice since it fosters an appreciation for food, rather than restricting your diet. It is healthy to have several food choices. Eating foods with varying textures, tastes, and flavors is healthy. Removing stress from eating is healthy. Enjoying your food is a crucial part of nourishing your body and soul, so a good experience with food is healthy.

The way you prepare your food has a lot to do with how you consume food. Preparing your food is part of the mindful eating experience as it creates appreciation and awareness. It gives you an opportunity to give thanks for nature's creation, and its ability to play a crucial role in your life. As you prepare and eat your food, you satisfy your physical hunger while paying attention to the nurturing qualities of eating in a healthy way. Learning to savor each bite creates a bond between your physical body, food, and your spirit.

Use the mindful eating practices daily, stay focused, and don't beat yourself up about small slip-ups. You have the power within you to change. Once you manifest your healthy eating into daily habits, you give yourself permission to enjoy food fully and without restrictions. These habits become a lifestyle that you can take with you wherever you go, and remain viable regardless of the obstacles you face. Make the decision to change your life today. Make the decision to be healthier and look after your body while eating what you want to eat.

***

Please leave a review for this book if you found the content useful.

If you enjoyed learning about Mindful Eating, but feel the concept is too vague for you, then you might find our other book useful. It is called *Intuitive Eating*. In this book, you will learn about intuitive eating, a similar concept to mindful eating, which has a lot more guidelines for eating healthily. It still allows you to eat what you want and remains a lifestyle plan rather than a diet.

YOUR FREE GIFTS

As a way of saying thanks for your purchase and to help you along your journey towards developing healthier eating habits, we've created free bonus resources that will help you get the best possible results:

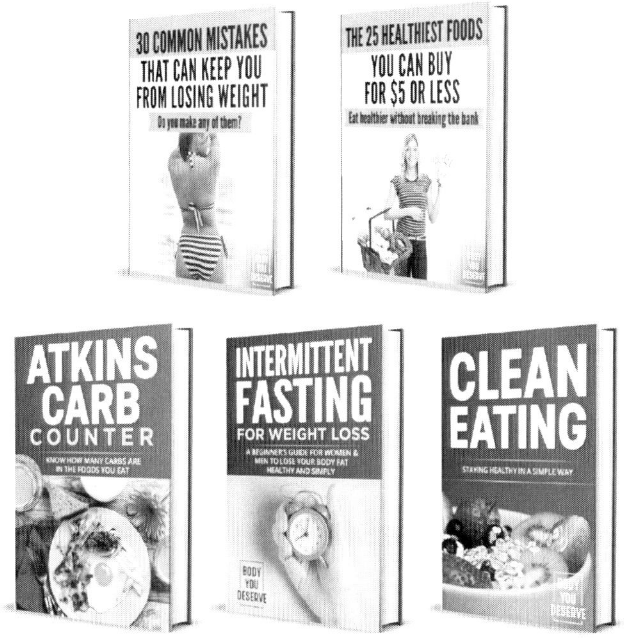

Free bonus #1: 30 Common mistakes that can keep you from losing weight
Do you make any of them?

Free bonus #2: The 25 Healthiest Foods You Can Buy for $5 or Less
Eat healthier without breaking the bank

Free bonus #3: Atkins carb counter
Know how many carbs are in the foods you eat

Free bonus #4: Intermittent Fasting for Weight Loss
A beginners guide for women & men to lose your body fat healthy and simply

Free bonus #5: Clean Eating
Staying healthy in a simple way

To get your bonuses, go to: http://bit.ly/NathalieSeaton

or scan with Your camera:

References

Ackerman, C.E. (2020). 58 Science-based mindful eating exercises and tips. Positive Psychology. https://positivepsychology.com/mindful-eating-exercises/

Ajmera, R. (n.d.). The effects of poor nutrition on your health. Live Strong. https://www.livestrong.com/article/31172-effects-poor-nutrition-health/

Albers, S. (2017). The surprising benefits of mindful eating. Huffpost. https://www.huffpost.com/entry/mindful-eating_b_1265865

Babauta, L. (n.d.). Dealing with emotional eating issues. Zen Habits. https://zenhabits.net/emotional-eating-issues/

Basso, J. C., McHale, A., Ende, V., Oberlin, D. J., & Suzuki, W. A. (2019). Brief, daily meditation enhances attention, memory, mood, and emotional regulation in non-experienced meditators. *Behav Brain Res. 1*(356), 208-220. https://pubmed.ncbi.nlm.nih.gov/30153464/

Bhandari, S. (2019). Why am I binge eating? WebMD. https://www.webmd.com/mental-health/eating-disorders/binge-eating-disorder/why-binge-eating#1

Bjarnadottir, A. (2019). Mindful eating 101. Healthline. https://www.healthline.com/nutrition/mindful-eating-guide

Chowles, E. (n.d.). Do you need to eat, want to eat, or feel like you should be eating? SleekGeek. https://www.sleekgeek.co.za/2019/02/do-you-need-to-eat-want-to-eat-or-feel-like-you-should-be-eating/

Cleveland Clinic. (2020). The psychology of eating. https://my.clevelandclinic.org/health/articles/10681-the-psychology-of-eating

Cleveland Clinic. (2020). Mindlessly snacking (again)? Try these simple mindful eating exercises. https://health.clevelandclinic.org/mindlessly-snacking-again-try-these-3-simple-mindful-eating-exercises/

Derbyshire Healthy Future Service. (n.d.). The hunger scale. http://www.dchs.nhs.uk/assets/public/dchs/llb//tools/tools_1-11/4_DCHS_A5_4pp_The_Hunger_Scale.pdf

DiR. (2019). 5 Risks and consequences of a poor diet. https://www.dir.cat/blog/en/risks-consequences-of-poor-diet/

Eddins, R. (2018). How to counter emotional eating with mindfulness. The Doctor Weighs In. https://thedoctorweighsin.com/how-to-counter-emotional-eating-with-mindfulness/

Everyday Health (n.d.). 9 Bad eating habits and how to break them. https://www.everydayhealth.com/diet-and-nutrition-pictures/bad-eating-habits-and-how-to-break-them.aspx

Fetters, K.A. (2015). 100 Things to do instead of eating mindlessly. Women's Health. https://www.womenshealthmag.com/weight-loss/a19902230/avoid-mindless-eating/

FitMind. (2020). Mindful eating: Science and exercise script. https://www.fitmind.co/blog-collection/mindful-eating-exercise-script

Godman, H. (2019). 11 Benefits of mindful eating. U.S. News. https://health.usnews.com/wellness/food/articles/benefits-of-mindful-eating

Halland, B. (2019). 6 Meditations to curb emotional eating. Thrive Global. https://thriveglobal.com/stories/6-meditations-to-curb-emotional-eating/

Hoge, E. A., Bui, E., Marques, L., Metcalf, C. A., Morris, L. K., Robinaugh, D. J., Worthington, J. J., Pollack, M. H., & Simon, N. M. (2013). Randomized controlled trial of mindfulness meditation for generalized anxiety disorder: Effects of anxiety and stress reactivity. *Journal of Clinical Psychiatry 74*(8), 786-792. https://www.ncbi.nlm.nih.gov/pmc/articles/PMC3772979/

Kirkpatrick, K. (2019). 7 Sneaky signs of an unhealthy diet. Cleveland Clinic. https://health.clevelandclinic.org/7-sneaky-signs-of-an-unhealthy-diet/
Kristeller, J. and Bowman, A. (2015). The joy of half a cookie: 9 principles that'll help you eat mindfully. The Mindful World. https://www.themindfulword.org/2015/principles-mindful-eating/
Malacoff, J. (2020). The science behind why eating is so comforting. MyFitnessPal. https://blog.myfitnesspal.com/the-science-behind-why-eating-is-so-comforting/
May, M. & Johnson, R. (n.d.). Mindful eating - Shifting the focus from weight to well-being. Corporate Wellness. https://www.corporatewellnessmagazine.com/article/mindful-eating-well-being
Mindfulness Exercises. (n.d.). Self kindness - part 1. https://mindfulnessexercises.com/self-kindness-part-1/
Monroe, J.T. (2015). Mindful eating: Principles and practice. American Journal of Lifestyle Medicine. https://journals.sagepub.com/doi/abs/10.1177/1559827615569682?journalCode=ajla#:~:text=The%20basic%20principles%20of%20mindful,to%20assist%20in%20achieving%20awareness.
Prichard, S. (2018). The many benefits of mindful eating. Skip Prichard. https://www.skipprichard.com/the-many-benefits-of-mindful-eating/
Rosenkranz, M. A., Davidson, R. J., MacCoon, D. G., Sheridan, J. F., Kalin, N. H., and Lutz, A. (2013). A comparison of mindfulness-based stress reduction and an active control in modulation of neurogenic inflammation. *Brain, Behavior, and Immunity 27*, 174-184. https://www.sciencedirect.com/science/article/abs/pii/S0889159112004758
Scott, J.R. (2020). What is binge eating? Very Well Mind. https://www.verywellmind.com/when-does-overeating-become-binge-eating-3495807
Smith, M., Robinson, L., Segal, J., & Segal, R. (2020). Emotional eating and how to stop it. HelpGuide. https://www.helpguide.org/articles/diets/emotional-eating.htm
Tamkin, T. (2019). Why science can't seem to tell us how to eat right. Nourish by WebMD. https://www.webmd.com/diet/news/20190422/why-science-cant-tell-us-how-to-eat-right
The Mindfulness Project. (2014). 3 Principles of mindful emotional eating. https://www.londonmindful.com/blog/3-principles-of-mindful-emotional-eating/
The Psych Professionals. (n.d.). Mindful Eating. https://psychprofessionals.com.au/mindful-eating/
Uotani, S. (2019). How to use mindfulness meditation to overcome emotional eating. BetterHumans. https://betterhumans.pub/how-to-use-mindfulness-meditation-to-overcome-emotional-eating-aa95003cfe64
Valentine, M. (n.d.). 20 Mindful eating tips that will transform your relationship with food. Buddhaimonia. https://buddhaimonia.com/blog/20-mindful-eating-tips
Wadyka, S. (2019). How mindful eating can help you lose weight. Consumer Reports. https://www.consumerreports.org/dieting-weight-loss/how-mindful-eating-can-help-you-lose-weight/
White, D.A. (2011). Top 10 worst eating habits. Food Network. https://www.foodnetwork.com/healthyeats/healthy-tips/2011/03/top-10-worst-eating-habits
The Art of Mindful Eating. (n.d.). The big five benefits of intuitive eating and eating mindfully. https://www.theartofmindfuleating.com/the-5-big-benefits-of-intuitive-eating-and-eating-mindfully/
Zelman, K.M. (n.d.). Why we eat the foods we do. Nourish by WebMD. https://www.webmd.com/diet/features/why-we-eat-the-foods-we-do#1

Intuitive Eating

A Revolutionary Program To Stop Dieting, Binging, Emotional Eating, Overeating and Feel Finally Free To Live the Life You Want

Introduction

What is the first thing that crossed your mind when you first picked up this book? Did you think, "Oh well, another diet that doesn't work," or "Will the food industry ever stop conning us?", or "Well, I might as well try this."

Whatever reasoning your mind came up with, we are sad to disclose that you are wrong! This book is nothing of the sorts.

If you are one of the 45 million Americans who have weight loss as their New Year Resolution then let us tell you, this isn't a weight loss book. Wait, don't just stop reading this, give us a chance to explain what it is if it is not a diet or weight loss book.

So, why did you pick up this book in the first place and how can it help you?

Chances are you picked it up because you haven't lost hope; hope in yourself and your relationship with food. If we were to do a psychic reading just now, we think you picked up this book because you are fed up with all your former diets and just wish there was something that can lead you to a normal and happy life where you didn't have to count every calorie in your food. Or maybe because you have spent the last 10 years of losing and gaining weight but failed to maintain it. Perhaps, you have just had a meal and you're still craving more. Maybe you picked up this book because you are obsessed with a certain food group say, desserts or beverages and you can't seem to stop. Or maybe you want to get out of binge and emotional eating patterns.

Whatever your reasons may be, let's get one thing clear, shall we?

This book isn't only about weight loss, it is also about eating healthy and nutritious food. It isn't about yo-yo dieting but rather a complete guide to embrace healthy eating behaviors. The purpose is to give you a break from dieting and help you start living your life like you should be. The goal is to allow you to see past a diet and experience what it feels like to have a diet-free life for once.

In this book, together we will go on a journey of a lifetime where not only will we tell you about intuitive eating but walk you through each step you need to take to become one. Talk about being a good partner!

With intuitive eating, you will learn how you can listen to your body's inner cues of hunger and fullness. With intuitive eating, you will realize that food can also be a source of pure joy and pleasure. With intuitive eating, you will reconnect with your body and honor it with the right nutrition. You will learn how to manage your cravings and recover from eating disorders.

You will learn about why you haven't been able to eat properly for as long as you can remember. You will learn that no matter how hard you try, chances are 95% of the diets will fail you. Don't believe us? Let us prove it to you right now!

You will also learn that diet culture is anything, but a myth and you certainly don't have to look a certain way to gain your partner's attention or a new suitor. Hell, ditch him if, even if it's one time, he tells you that you need to change who you are!

Once you are done doing that, come back to read more about how this is going to be a revolutionary change, maybe not as big as the Apollo 11 to Mars, but no less for someone with a bad relationship with food.

So, are you all set for the biggest change of your life?

Yes!

Say it louder, we can't hear you.

Yes!!

Louder than that...

Yes!!!

Wow let's begin then!

Chapter 1: The Act of Eating

In this first chapter, we are going to be talking about the science of food, how we choose amongst different foods, what factors differentiate between the food we like and don't like, why we eat the way we do — sometimes in three meals and sometimes six — why we keep failing at diets or more precisely, why do they keep failing us, what kind of eater you are.

Interesting, no? Well, how about we make it more interesting with some amazing research work over the years to determine the likelihood of you picking an apple instead of an orange. You may not realize this but there is a ton going on behind this decision of yours and we are going to break it down for you below.

Why Do We Eat the Foods We Eat?

It isn't as simple as we eat because we are hungry. In his book tilted *Mindless Eating: Why We Eat More Than We Think*, Dr. Brian Wansink, a renowned food psychologist studied the consumption patterns of humans and why they eat the way they do. According to Wansink, we unintentionally make about 200 food decisions every single day! However, we aren't even aware of 90% of them. We are going to be looking at some more thought-provoking studies found in his book to help us understand better.

Cravings for Bad Food

One of the key features of nearly every diet ever created involves complete abstinence from some food. Sometimes, it is bad carbs, proteins or even dairy! This is where the fault lies. Human psychologists suggest that the more we are told to abstain from something the more we crave it. So, now you know why it is so hard to put that big slice of cake back in the fridge. This behavior is even prevalent in kids. How many times did you tell little Jimmy to not put his finger in the socket? Does he stop? Yeah, we know!

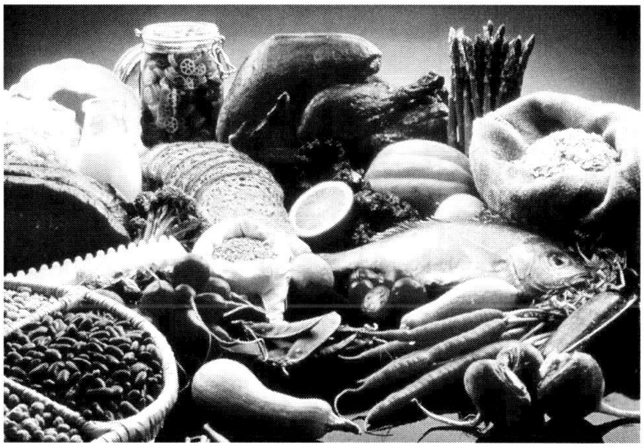

So basically, every time someone tells you that you need to stay away from something when you are trying to shed a few pounds, they are setting you up for cravings for that exact same thing.

Cheap Vs. Expensive

According to another study that put all the wine experts to shame is the difference between the expensive and cheap wine conducted by a Ph.D. student named Frederic Brochet at the University of Bordeaux (Morrot, Brochet, & Dubourdieu, 2001).

In the experiment, Frederic argued that the branding of what we buy has a lot to do with the perception we have of it in our minds. In his study, he gathered 57 participants and served them with a red Bordeaux from a midrange bottle with a label that referred to it as a modest vin de table.

The same participants were called back a week later to try another bottle of red Bordeaux from a high-end bottle with a label that termed it as grand cru. The participants were then asked to rate their experience of the first wine and the second. A majority of them rated the first wine as weak, unbalanced, and simple. The second wine from a different label was rated as complex and balanced. The most shocking thing was that the wine in both bottles had been similar. Frederic called this perspective the expectation that most of us have towards certain brands. Although they are serving the exact same thing, we tend to believe that they are somehow better than the competition since they are expensive and look more sophisticated.

Here's another crazy study in which the researchers asked some participants to try out a cup of flavored yogurt but in a dark room. The researchers had specifically told the participants that the yogurt was chocolate flavored even though it wasn't. It was strawberry flavored.

Surprisingly, 59% of the participants rated the chocolate-flavored yogurt as having a mild and subtle strawberry flavor that they loved the most. So you see, just because they were told something all along, their minds tricked them into thinking it was.

This is what the marketing industry is built upon. Breeding that very perception in our minds that despite knowledge, we tend to overlook the obvious and give in. This is also how most of your favorite celebrities are earning viewers when marketing diets, makeup or beauty treatments. They assure you that you need them to look better and more like them, which isn't true.

Presentation Matters the Most!

Be it in Master Chef or your favorite restaurant, a lot of times it comes down to how well a dish has been presented even if it is as simple as mashed potatoes or a slice of cake. The art of presentation does have a positive impact on our brains and boost hunger.

This very phenomenon was studied in this next research where the experimenters presented brownies in three different ways (Grabinsky, et al., 2015). However, everyone was getting the same brownies to taste. It was just the presentation that differed. Participants were divided into three different groups.

- The first group was presented brownies in a china dish.
- The second group was presented brownies on a paper plate.
- The third group was presented brownies on a tissue paper.

The experimenters then asked the participants how much they will be willing to pay for the brownies.

- The first group said that they would pay $1.27 for each piece of brownie.
- The second group said that they would pay 76 cents for each piece of brownie.
- The third group said that they would pay 53 cents for each piece of brownie.

This means that the presentation does have an appeal on our brain and purchasing. No wonder we always go for the shiniest thing in the store just because it seems more tempting to have.

Who Wants a Hershey's Kiss?

In an experiment, Wansink conducted on the secretaries in an office. He found that when they sat near a clear dish of Hershey's kisses in comparison to an opaque dish filled with the same, they ate more. Furthermore, they gained five extra pounds over the year. It was calculated that secretaries sitting near a clear dish of Hershey's kisses consumed 77 calories a day (Wansink, 2005).

The point, in case, was that whenever something is placed in front of us, we tend to incline towards it, even when we aren't hungry. The presence of it tricks the mind into thinking that it is craving for it. And it happens with everyone. Whether it is a boxful of donuts in a police station or a bag of chips in your lounge, if you see it, you are likely to eat it.

Up for Some Popcorn, Anyone?

Another interesting experiment in the book also reveals that when we are given a large portion of something, we eat more. Yes, we are talking about that hearty steak meal you get at your favorite diner with a side of mashed potatoes and veggies. In a study, Wansink gave some moviegoers the choice to opt for a medium or a large size of popcorn tub. Despite saying that the size didn't matter, moviegoers with the larger tub of popcorn ate 53% more than those with a smaller tub. This proved that when we are presented with something in large quantities, we eat more of it, even if we aren't able to finish it all.

Why Do We Eat the Way We Do?

Coming to the second important aspect of why we eat the way we do, many researchers believe that our age, gender, lifestyle, family history, and hormones have a lot to do with that. Published in the *Journal of American College of Nutrition*, the IFIC Foundation research aimed to identify the factors that impacted on the way we eat so that we can understand how we can make changes and adapt to better and healthier lifestyles.

The research discussed what exactly we wish to achieve when we eat the things we do and whether it changes with our age, gender or body mass index (BMI).

Approximately 2,700 American adults participated in an online survey from age 18-80. The survey was demographically charted and consisted of 6,689 drinking and eating occasions the participants reported during the day before.

Astonishing results surfaced which defied the previous assumptions about how we eat, how often we consume food and drinks, and why we preferred them over the others. It was believed that the decision to eat had to do with the lifestyle characteristics of the participants. Age was another important factor that helped the researchers understand why we eat the way we do. Seniors were more likely to plan their meals as per schedule than adults and teenagers. It showed that they used the time of the day as a trigger rather than hunger itself. If they had lunch at 12:00 am every day, they resorted to that time only.

Secondly, it was also believed that moderation in eating and drinking also contributed to why we eat the way we do. The respondents stopped eating when they felt satisfied, had enough, or when their plate was empty. However, this moderation differed for every individual.

If we take this research as a beacon of guidance, we realize that the reason we eat isn't entirely based on hunger but rather motivated by factors like the presence of food, time or habit. This can help those trying to manage their weight as they can focus on the factors that trigger eating and thus avoid them.

What Kind of Eater Are You?

Now, here's the next important thing. What kind of eater are you determines what practices you adopt when it comes to eating. Do you confide by time or are you walking with a spoon in your pocket all the time? Do you prefer a proper setting or any place is good for you as long as you get something to eat? Are there any restaurants you prefer for hygiene basis or do you base your food choices solely on taste? All these questions will help you understand your eating habits and whether they need to change or not.

Confused? Keep reading and you will understand what we are talking about.

Emotional Eater

Are you someone who, every time watches The Notebook cries with a pint of Ben and Jerry's in your bed? Are you someone who eats just because they are bored and have nothing else to do? Do you treat yourself with a drink every time you finish a report before its due date out of sheer happiness?

If all these sound like things you do, you are an emotional eater. You are someone who eats according to their mood and not their hunger. You celebrate with a bottle of whiskey and dig your spoon into ice-cream when you're sad. All your eating habits revolve around how you feel. There isn't much care for rational thinking before you pick something up. This often leads to eating more when you see your weight creeping and being unable to fit into your skinny jeans. The cycle goes on and on until you move to hazardous and stringent diets that do you more harm than good. An emotional eater just eats to satisfy themselves.

Critical Eater

A critical eater is someone who either has set preferences on what they eat or nothing at all. They are an all-or-nothing kind of individual. Critical eaters are obsessed with diets despite knowing the nutritional importance. They usually have a hard time sticking to just one diet as they expect fast changes. When they don't happen as per their set goals, they give up and move onto the next one. They have this preset notion that dieting makes them a conscious and good human being which means that when they are not on one, they consider themselves as bad. They give in to the temptations of delicacies but regret it later by going on strict and restrictive diets that sometimes has consequences.

Habitual Eater

As the name suggests, a habitual eater is someone who indulges in bad food choices, giving themselves the excuse that they will only try it once. They know the importance of eating right, maintenance of an eating routine and preferences, but sometimes, they are derailed by responsibilities and time constraints. One of the biggest disadvantages of being a habitual eater is that habitual eaters don't eat when they feel their appetite building, instead, they eat because they are used to it. They might say something like, "I will have dinner by 7:00 p.m. and not a minute late. After dinner, I will not eat anything till the next morning." This mentality of eating at a fixed time prevents them from listening to their internal cues.

Energy Eater

Imagine someone with a granola bar in their hands as their breakfast and they can't shut up about the benefits it holds. Yes, we all have that one colleague in our office or a friend in our social circle. Energy eaters are all about quick fixes. You will always find them talking about the nutritional facts of things and their favorite, on-the-go snacks throughout the day. The only problem, however, is that they eat too much of them. Although there isn't any harm in eating energy fixing food, an excess of it can be counterintuitive. A majority of energy bars and foods come packed with calories that our bodies may not require. In fact, sometimes, instead of trying to eat healthily and consume fewer fatty foods to avoid calories, we eat more of them found in granola bars. Besides, they also increase insulin production in the body, which isn't good for your overall health and leads to making you feel hungrier.

External Eater

External eaters wait for external cues to eat. Oh, it's a colleague's birthday? Bring in the cake. Oh, it's a baby shower, let's get your hands full with the sugary delights placed so elegantly on a platter. Such external cues trigger their hunger and not their body. Their brain awaits for such signals to occur so it can trigger hunger. These people are the worst to hang out with as they will stop at every cupcake shop or roadside hot dog stall because they are tempted to eat. This can result in overeating without the eater even realizing and later suffering from digestive issues and complaining about it to you.

Sensual Eater

A sensual or mindful eater appreciates whatever is presented in front of them. They don't just eat the food, they devour all the flavors and spices in it sensually. They will moan at how juicy that steak is, they will give a shout out to the waiter for the delicious wine, and later leave a thank you note for the chef who made the red velvet cake. The point here is that they love to explore the food involving all their senses. They are in no rush to finish up and chug everything down, instead; they relish in the exploration and deliciousness of it. Unlike critical or picky eaters, they don't always think about making rational decisions when it comes to food.

Chaotic Eater

A chaotic eater is someone who will eat whatever they can whenever they can. They skip meals frequently and usually eat on the run. They also have little memory of what they ate or when which means they either starve their bodies or overeat. They don't plan or schedule their meals and don't have any specific preferences either. This usually results in them gaining or losing weight overtime — both of which impact their overall well-being and health over time.

Restrictive Eater

A restrictive eater is also similar to a critical eater as they are very particular about the food they eat. They are mostly on diets and have journals listing their calorie intake for every meal. They also follow a strict choice of food and have a list of items they can and can't eat. They don't give in to the temptation of what lies in front of them. If you know of someone who is a restrictive eater, you may have spotted them weighing their meals, reading labels of products and charting them. Since they are so strict about their food options, they often fear eating food prepared by others or with others. Even before they are finished with their current meal, they start worrying about their next one.

Intuitive Eater

Intuitive eaters are different from any of the eaters mentioned above. They wait for physical cues from their bodies. They don't indulge in mindless eating and only eat when their body tells them too. They rarely give in to temptations. They also look for cues to stop eating to prevent overeating. They experience no guilt and have trust in themselves when they are around food. But this doesn't mean they don't enjoy their food because they do as there are no restrictions about what to eat or how much to eat.

Take Away

In this chapter, we take a look at our connection with food, what motivates or stops us when it comes to choosing between different food groups. Later, we also discuss why we eat the way we do and how sticking to a fixed schedule to eating is doing us more harm than good and why the practice must be made obsolete. Finally, we tried to categorize people into different categories of eating from restrictive eater to an intuitive eater.

Chapter 2: Intuitive Eating – The Program to Quit All Diets

Researchers at the University of California published a report in the 2017's edition of the *Journal of American Psychologist* which aimed to understand and monitor the long-term effects of dieting. The study proposed that 66.6% of dieters didn't lose weight over five years dieting all the way and in some cases even gained more weight. Whenever we come across such statistics, they reinforce the idea that conventional diets may offer desirable results for the short-term, but they aren't the way of life. The restriction to certain foods and the addition of others only causes a misbalance. This is where intuitive eating comes in.

What Is Intuitive Eating?

A term or phenomenon coined by two Californian nutritionists Evelyn Tribole and Elyse Resch; the intuitive eating program is listening to your body's innate need for food. It involves biological wisdom that each of us possesses but fail to pay heed to. According to the originators, our body already knows what food and nutrients it requires. It also knows when to eat, when to stop, and the best habits to adopt concerning food. It is a better judge by miles in comparison to the dietary recommendations that the majority of the diets and its practitioners rub in our faces.

Intuitive eating program steers away from rigid dietary requirements and scientific explanations and lays value to the psychological need for eating. When we begin to eat intelligently, we try to find that lost inner wisdom and let it guide us to ensure that our body remains healthy and well-fed.

What led to the discovery of the idea were conventional dietary programs. The developers of the idea questioned why diets failed to work. It was thought-provoking that despite the many conventional diets available in the markets, Americans weren't losing weight. The obesity rate in the country continued to rise. Furthermore, the developers also discovered that dieting had a major consequence which they termed the diet backlash. The diet backlash refers to an observation that dieting for many years led to multiple eating disorders and promoted guilty, compulsive, binging, and self-loathing behaviors in many. This was because whilst diets promoted the usage of certain foods, it also asked the dieters to restrict from some. The restrictive foods were of course more delectable and crave-able, which only led to frustration upon rejecting it and guilt upon giving in to its temptation.

To further prove the point that intuitive eating was true, the only suitable way, the originators cited a 1991 study by Dr. Leann Birch. It was published in the *New England Journal of Medicine* and revolved around the eating habits of children. According to the research's findings, children have the innate ability to regulate their habits around eating. They can also do so in a healthy manner. This meant that parental control over what they should eat and what they shouldn't was in fact, counterproductive. Some other studies also confirm that the additional pressure from parents to eat right has led to bulimia, anorexia and other eating disorders in teenagers and children. This is a common sight to behold in participants taking part in beauty pageants from an early age. They are made to follow a strict diet and denied all pleasures of what being a kid comes with. In some studies, it has also led to issues with self-esteem and self-loathing. Coming back to the original study, if the children do possess that innate wisdom to eating right, there must be some way to rekindle it within them as they grow older and allow it to blossom so that healthy choices can be made.

Lastly, the originators of the intuitive eating program also registered that no matter how well-conceived a diet is, it only has short-term implications. This isn't the case with intuitive eating. In fact, intuitive eating shuns all such beliefs that dieting is good for you and encourage you to listen to your body's needs and accept the way you look. It also promotes the health movement and strongly believes that health conditions like poor dietary habits and obesity leads to increased risk of diseases and illnesses.

So, if we were to summarize the hyped concept of eating intuitively, we have the following four domains.

Relying on Satiety Cues

The first crucial area in an intuitive eating program is to establish trust in your innate hunger and wait for the satiety cues. Let these cues guide your eating behavior. How does it differ from conventional dietary restraints? It differs in the way we let our internal cues determine our eating regimes instead of our external cues. For instance, the majority of diets propose that one must break down meals into five to six smaller meals per day. However, there is no such limitation in eating intuitively. You must eat when you feel hungry and how much you should eat must depend on your calorie-burning capacity and metabolic rate.

Quitting to Eat for Emotional Reasons

Secondly, in intuitive eating, you look for the physical reasons for eating rather than solely relying on your mood or emotions. Intuitive eating implies that one must only eat when their body shows physical signs of hunger such as a growling stomach and also stop when it feels full. This disregards two very important notions with diets, for example, overeating and eating because you are overwhelmed with emotions.

You Don't Need Permission to Eat

Unlike most fad diets that clock your meals, there is no such concept in intuitive eating. This domain involves your willingness to eat whenever hungry and refusing to label foods as good or bad. When you eat as per your own body's schedule and needs, you prevent overindulgence and the shame and guilt accompanying it.

Not Categorizing your Food

In this last but important domain regarding intuitive eating, you begin to realize that every food has a purpose to serve. Be it any vegetable, fruit or protein, each has its own benefits for our bodies and must be taken without restrictions. However, the context of the situation may vary.

The Psychology of Eating Intuitively

Imagine waking up in a world where your relationship with food was easy. You ate the things you love, at whatever time you felt hungry, stopped eating when you're full and leading an active and healthy life. Alas, in the real world, it isn't this easy. So, who has made it difficult?

You!

Yes, it is you who has made the eating process so calculative, restrictive, and scheduled. Imagine if you continued to eat the way you are supposed to, there wouldn't have been any moments of guilt or being hard on yourself. There wouldn't have been any beating yourself up later when your stomach got upset or you put on weight. There wouldn't have been any eating linked to how you felt — happy, sad, angry or stressed.

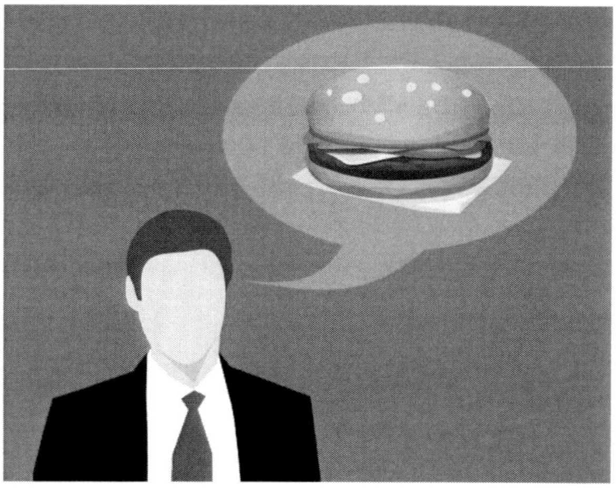

Think about just eating for the sake of eating and providing your body with the nutrients and energy it requires. Is it that hard?

Not really.

Believe it or not, but the picture we presented at the start of this section can be your reality if you want it to be. Your relationship with food should be based on trust. You should be able to trust your body to signal your cues when to eat and trusting it to tell you when to stop. Once you begin to make well-informed decisions regarding your food, you won't have to rely on fad diets anymore.

But how does it actually work and what is the psychology behind it?

Intuitive eating is a scientifically proven phenomenon. It works, in the same manner our inner gut works. Have you ever had déjà vu or feeling like something wasn't right? Perhaps, you are walking down a dark alley and feel like someone is stalking you? Or felt your heart beating faster when you are with a loved one or meet your favorite celebrity for the first time? Ever had that uncomfortable pinching in your stomach when you didn't feel sure about something? Have you ever gotten all sweaty and shaking when you're going for a job interview?

What is it if it's not your body's enteric nervous system signaling you? Science refers to it as our gut-brain. Odd, but we do have a brain in our belly too. This gut-brain differs from the brain we have in our heads but works in the same manner, more or less. The enteric nervous system lies in between the muscle layers of the esophagus, small intestine, and the stomach just under the mucosal lining. There is a complex network of neurochemicals and neurons that help teleport any messages and signals our gut-brain is suggesting.

Researchers believe that our enteric nervous system is constantly throwing out suggestions and giving information about your nutritional needs to the brain. However, since we are so used to listening to the external cues, we often miss hearing it. Think about it, how many of us eat when the lunch hour begins? Or when our parents call us down because the dinner is served? Or when we are hanging out with friends or a partner to dine out? The first rule of eating intuitively is listening to the internal messages and honoring and trusting them to make decisions regarding your food.

Why We Fear Listening to Our Gut-Brain?

If listening to your gut-brain is as easy as paying attention to a speaker in a seminar, why can't we all do it? There are a few fears involved.

For starters, most of us believe that by listening to our inner cues to tell us what we should eat and how much, we might resort to unhealthy eating behaviors and end up making the wrong choices. Who knows if we are decoding the signals the right way? What if we end up overeating and gaining weight over time? This sounds sensible but it is also bad judgment. This arises from the lack of trust we have in our body and the natural cues it is capable to give us. But you can't be blamed for it entirely either. We have been brought up this way and it is hard to give up after so many years, isn't it ladies? Of course, regaining trust with your relationship with food involves just you, and it can seem hard. If only there were some counselors to guide us through the process and rekindle that lost spark. Okay, maybe we went a little off-road here.

Coming back to our original point, it will take time to rebuild trust in your body and take an ounce of patience on your part. But it is worth it in the end. If you stick to it forever, you will never have to go back to dieting again.

The worst thing about any diet is that it promotes the elimination of some foods. However, did you ever realize that the foods you aren't allowed to eat are also the ones you crave the most? And what's even worse is that you didn't even want them before you started the diet. For instance, let's say you don't have a sweet tooth. You come across a diet that restricts any sugar content. You think to yourself, "Great, I don't even like sweets that much. This would be so much easier to pick." A week down the lane and you see this stunning layered chocolate lava cake in the hands of a waiter serving it to a couple next to your table in a restaurant and you feel something within you. What's that? A craving? But you didn't feel this way when you saw a chocolate cake before. Then why all of a sudden you want to fork it down your tummy? Somehow you still resist the temptation and tell yourself that once you are done with the diet, this will be the first thing you will have. And you do! In fact, you overindulge in it, having it more often than before. And then in no time, you see the dropped pounds creeping back up and you are right back to where you started.

It is very natural for your body to crave the things it has been restricted from. The longer you put it off, the more intense your cravings will become.

With intuitive eating, there is no restriction which means no cravings. Every food is allowed and thus, feels normal. When you reach this point where you stop experiencing sudden cravings, you are on the path to becoming an intuitive eater. It is important to understand that cravings don't always happen for fast food, carbs, and sugary delights. It can even happen for the simplest of foods. Picture this, you are traveling to a different country on vacation. You are excited to try the local cuisine. You do and for some time you find it tantalizing as well. But after some days or perhaps weeks, you will miss the cuisine from your country. You will be surprised that you will be craving for food you called boring and sad and hated when it was made it your home. So basically, we just don't crave the things we can't have but also the things we do, and it all comes down to having a variety of everything. This is what intuitive eating programs preach.

They tell you to listen to your body's hunger cues and what it is craving. When everything is consumed in a natural and limited manner, your body will resort to a weight that feels normal. This is referred to as the body's set-point weight. Let us help you understand it with a very basic example. Imagine you placed water in a container and kept it out. When you first kept it, it was at room temperature. If the weather outside in the daytime is sunny and warm, the water's temperature will increase after a few hours. During the night, the weather changes and it becomes chilly. The water's temperature will decrease. Hunger and metabolism operate in the same manner.

Hunger cues and metabolism plays a crucial role in our body's regulation of weight. We only feel hunger when our weight falls beyond our set-point weight. Metabolism also slows down in case energy is required. However, when we feed ourselves and feel full, our set-point weight goes up and the rate of metabolism increases to bring the body back to its set-point weight.

How to Eat Intuitively: A Step-by-Step Guide to Prepare Yourself

Now that we have covered the majority of what intuitive eating is all about, it is time we actually learn how to implement it in our lives to start listening to our body's natural responses and maintaining a healthy weight without having to give up on something. We have broken it down into six simple steps to get you into the intuitive eating mode and prepare yourself for a better change in your lifestyle.

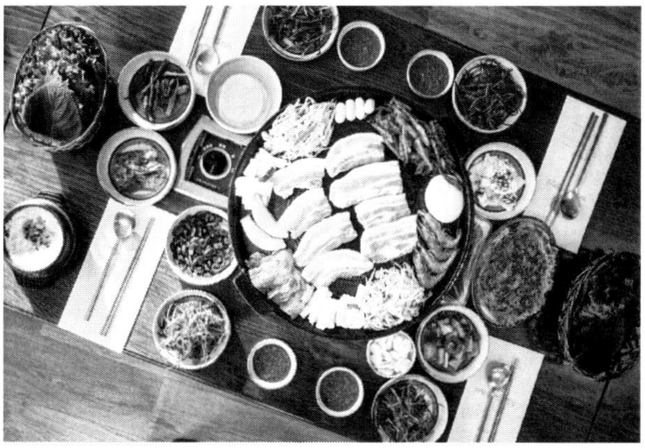

1. **Have Realistic Expectations and Accept the Way You Look**

First things first, we are all beautiful in the eyes of our loved ones. People who really love us, love us for who we are including the way we look. Besides, we were born to stand out and thanks to our unique genetic blueprint, we do! Then why do we always want to join the crowd and become invisible? Doesn't sound too ideal, does it, ladies?

So, if you have a few extra pounds hanging around your waist or have a double chin, that doesn't necessarily mean you aren't healthy, or you need to change the way you look. Of course, change is a requisite when your chubbiness gets in the way of your health and increases your risk of certain diseases. If not, then there is no reason to keep trying to reach an unsustainable, unrealistic and unhealthy weight.

You need to set realistic goals and expectations when starting with intuitive eating. Since it isn't like most diets, you are less likely to observe the results overnight. Setting the bar too high for yourself will only sadden you later when you fail to hit the mark. Besides, a good eating habit shouldn't involve stress and harm to your self-worth. You need to be accepting of the way you look and stop beating yourself about it. The sooner you let go of the guilt that makes you want to try on different diets every now and then, the better off you will be — physically and emotionally.

2. **Understand That Fad Diets Aren't Going to Work**

If your main concern is to lose weight, it may seem tempting to pick a diet that promises guaranteed and quick results. However, this weight loss is usually temporary and comes with many drastic measures such as radically cutting down calories, eliminating food groups or sticking to low-carb diets only. Since these measures are quite challenging and directly attacking the body's natural biology, they lead to cravings in the long run. Moreover, there is always a chance of falling off the wagon and feeling guilty and self-doubt.

So, the more rational thing to do here is to rely on a food routine that has worked for people for centuries and includes eating real food in moderation and moving around. When preparing to eat intuitively, you must look for nutrient-enriched diets that promise steady energy levels, a stable mind, and a healthy body. You must choose foods that honor your health. You must eat things that satisfy your hunger and taste buds and make you feel good and energetic.

3. Shun the Good or Bad Thinking About Food

Some foods are more nutrient-dense than others but that doesn't mean you should eliminate them completely from your diet. Doing so will only add to your stress levels of not having that forbidden food and increase your craving for it. If you are trying to become an intuitive eater, you need to make peace with food, stop fighting, and settle for a truce. Now, this doesn't mean that you go all out on processed goods because that is what you crave. You still need to prioritize foods that are healthy. However, you can always have them in limited quantities if the craving doesn't go away.

If you keep telling yourself that you need to abstain from certain food groups completely, it will also lead to feelings of shame and guilt in case you end up breaking your vows. Researchers believe that a mentality of all or nothing gives rise to binge eating. Those who give in to the temptation of their craving often end up having more of it and later regret their decision.

Your goal shouldn't be to strive for perfection here, but rather progress. Consistently eating healthy should be the ultimate goal without having to give up on your favorite comfort foods. Moreover, you need to stop labeling food groups as good or bad or black or white. You need to establish a balance between the two and aim to have more of the healthier foods than the unhealthy ones. This way you won't have to feel guilty about having your favorite foods or eating them in large quantities.

4. Eat When You're Hungry, Stop When You're Full

We have already discussed this several times above that intuitive eating promotes eating when your body asks for it and then stopping when it is full. There isn't any room for overeating or eating out of habit if you are trying to become an intuitive eater. This will also help you honor the food in front of you as you feel blessed to have it and discourage overeating or overindulgence. When you make this a habit, you will begin to notice that you will no longer crave food and only eat when your body tells you to.

5. Don't Use Food to Handle Your Emotions and Stress

Yes, we understand, there is hardly anything more satisfying than downing a whole cheesecake while watching Bridget Jones Diary because you feel like that is you. Just because of a bad date, breakup or anxiety due to a tough and unappreciated work life, you can't always go to food for comfort.

Emotional eating may seem like the best choice, but it is only going to make your situation worse. How so? Because then you would also have to deal with the guilt and shame that creeps up after you are done with your comfort food and have a stomachache. If you are wondering what should be the alternative, then you already know where this is going. Eat intuitively!

For a majority of people, eating intuitively opens doors to new possibilities to deal with stress without resorting to fatty, oily or carbs-dense foods. If you are looking for means to cope up with your stress and emotions in a healthy manner, start an intuitive eating journal or download intuitive eating apps that are readily available in the market today. Jotting down the amount of food you eat, how you felt after its consumption, and how many calories it has can all take off some stress and guilt that usually builds up when you don't eat intuitively.

6. **Fill Yourself with Sufficient Calories**

Got a bridal shower to attend or is it a high school reunion? We get it, you want to look your best and those few extra pounds you put on over the holidays are just adding to your anxiety. Of course, you want to lose them but resorting to temporary quick-fixes and fad diets aren't the solution. Experts believe that when we suddenly deprive our bodies of say, calories, it lowers our energy levels and slows down our metabolism. And the pounds you shed will come back in less time it took you to lose it because it will be mostly water weight. So, it may seem like it will work short-term but with consequences that can and will be long-term. Depriving your body in such a way will make you fatigued, stressed out, and feeling discontent.

How Is It Different from Mindful Eating?

A lot of people who are new to intuitive eating think of mindful eating and intuitive eating as the same. Although they can't be used synonymously, there are several similarities between the two. Some researchers go as far as suggesting that neither can exist without the other. Then why the different names and different approaches?

In this section, we are going to be looking at the many similarities and differences between the two and then let you decide if these two works in unison or not.

Starting with the similarities:

- Both mindful eating and intuitive eating are approaches to eating without the concept of dieting. They both strongly believe that the diet culture must be eliminated, and healthy eating should be promoted.
- Secondly, they both encourage forming a healthy relationship with food and not simply eat for the sake of eating but rather enjoying and seeking pleasure from it.

- Thirdly, they both have been used as a tool for weight loss and proven effective in the long-term.
- And lastly, there is no judgment when it comes to what you are eating or how much you are eating. The goal of both these approaches is simply to promote the consumption of the healthiest, nutrient-dense foods to lead a healthy lifestyle.

Although there aren't any major ones, the subtle differences between the two include:

- Where mindful eating opens your curiosity and encourages you to notice and appreciate the food in front of you, intuitive eating is more concerned with your body's needs.
- Where mindful eating can sometimes be used as a tool to measure and limit how much you eat, there is no such restriction with intuitive eating. Intuitive eating allows you to eat to your heart's content and be a little mindless about it.
- Where mindful eating preaches open-mindedness, intuitive eating is more about rejecting the diet mentality and culture.

Take Away

In this chapter, we covered the basics of what intuitive eating is all about, why we should adopt intuitive eating, the science behind it and a step by step guide for beginners planning to get started. Next, we addressed a common misconception about intuitively eating where many people thought it was synonymous with mindful eating. Therefore, we compiled a list of all the similarities and differences to help the readers distinguish between the changes and understand intuitive eating more aptly.

Chapter 3: The Principles of Intuitive Eating

Have you ever wondered why we adapt to the diet culture? What made us rely so much on them that we are willing to sacrifice our basic body's needs for it? It all started when our parents strictly told us to finish everything on our plates. Leaving even a pea behind was never an option whether we were hungry or not. We were told to drink milk and abstain from sweets. In fact, some parents didn't even allow their kids to devour the candy they collected on Halloween. We were then told that some foods were good for us as they helped us grow and some were bad and must be avoided. When all that happened, we stopped listening to the internal cues from our bodies and listened to the external ones instead. Society is to blame as it taught us how much we should eat, what we should eat, and what to avoid. Had it not been this coercing, we might have had a completely different looking body and health.

The ten principles of intuitive eating discard this notion and list down ways we can have a healthy relationship with our food and body. Let's take a look at what they are and how we can incorporate them into our lives to live a fulfilling and diet-free life.

1. Reject the Diet Mentality

Did you know that 95% of diets fail? But if we are going to be talking about the failure of diets, it is crucial to understand that it isn't the diet that fails, but the people who fail at diets. There is a vast difference between the two. Research has shown that dieting for a long period can have drastic consequences on our health and well-being. Since most diets expect their followers to go against their biological needs, it often leads to you questioning about your internal intuition. Moreover, every new diet somehow affects our level of confidence as well and is accompanied by guilt when we fail to keep going. This sets in feelings of unworthiness where you feel like you are an outcast and a disgrace to your own self and society.

Thus, when you reject the diet mentality, you free yourself from all the fatigue, shaming, obsession, yo-yo, and failure. And the best part, it isn't very hard to adopt either.

How to Reject the Diet Mentality?

Here's how you can reject the diet mentality and move towards a diet-free and guilt-free eating lifestyle.

- **Identify what really is the diet mentality**

It often feels like the entire fitness and wellness industry is making money off your insecurities and imperfections, doesn't it? They target the weaker ones and urge them to spend hundreds if not thousands of dollars into fixing themselves. In today's world, obsession and idolization regarding your health have become a norm. You don't even realize that you are surrounded by it completely and falling into its trap one step at a time. It is high time that you see it for what it is and recognize that you don't need to be a part of it. You are better off without it and not going to lose your hard earned money to the big corporations.

- **Distance yourself from things that promote diet mentality**

Since the goal is to eliminate this culture the first thing that you need to do is distance yourself from all those things that encourage dieting in the first place. This involves unfollowing all those diet accounts, people, and celebrities on social media like Facebook or Instagram who post their everyday routine workout sessions and diet plans and talk about all those expensive products, supplements, and training they used to look the way they do!

Secondly, unsubscribe to all those email reminders that pop up suggesting a sale on a weightless supplement and how you can save money by buying a year's worth supply. You don't need that.

Thirdly, unfriend all those people who constantly put you down over the way you look. Nobody has the right to tell you what you should do, eat or what you should wear. Your body is your temple and only you get to decide what it needs.

- **Learn about the long-term dangers of dieting**

We have linked several studies in the previous chapters that suggest that dieting does more harm than good. Take note of those studies and educate yourself. Let your mind make a rational decision about what is good and what isn't.

Dieting is one of the many reasons that lead to binge eating. Ever been to a party where you just can't put your spoon down and keep asking for seconds? If so, that is what dieting does to you. You overeat and purge on food.

2. Honor Your Hunger

The second principle demands that you honor your hunger. What does that actually mean?

Honoring your hunger means that you wait for the cues your body will most likely signal when it's time to eat. By honoring your food, you teach your body to eat not only foods that are available but also foods that it is asking for. For instance, if you feel like indulging in a big cheesy burger, don't try to shrug off the need with something else. Instead, have that burger and let your body know that you will continue to nourish and honor its needs as long as they are sensible and healthy. This involves building a trusting relationship with your food and body.

How to Honor Your Hunger?

- **Educate Yourself About What Hunger Feels Like**

There are several ways hunger is felt by someone. Sometimes, it is that growling feeling you get in your stomach which feels as if someone is twisting it. Other times, it is that lightheadedness that suggests that you are running low on energy. Then there is abdominal pain, irritability, fatigue, inability to concentrate, weakness or preoccupation with food. All these are cues that our body uses to remind us that we need to eat.

However, if you still aren't sure that you are getting mixed signals from your body, track your time with food. It takes about an average of 4-6 hours for your body to digest food. This means that you should feel hungry after 4-6 hours. But this isn't set in stone as our bodies are different from one another. Also, it depends on what you have consumed in your last meal as some foods take longer to digest.

- **Calculate Your Hunger and Fullness Scale**

Since we all feel and express hunger in different ways, it is only fair that we all have our personalized hunger and fullness scales. A hunger and fullness scale is a scale with two extremes. Think of it as a 1 to 10 scale where 1 represents most hungry and 10 most full. You need to rank your hunger and fullness based on these figures. If you are at one, you are starving to death and if you are at 10, you can't take another bite of your food.

Ideally, your hunger and fullness scale should range from 4 to 7. This way, you are eating before you are too starved and finishing before being physically full. Remaining in the in between will eliminate the physical discomforts such as lightheadedness or bloating and gas when you're too full.

Feed Your Body What It Is Asking For

When you feed your body the sustenance it wants, you are building body trust. However, if you still wish to remain on the healthier side of the spectrum, the best way is to keep foods that are healthy in your pantry and fridge. Another way to do so is to prep your meals in advance so your body already knows what it's going to get in a few hours and will most likely crave that.

The ultimate goal should be to honor your hunger. This means that if your body is craving cake, don't try to substitute it with a cookie just because you think it would be unhealthy. That is cheating and not honoring your hunger.

3. Make Peace with Food

This next principle allows you to consume all the food groups in your repertoire without penalizing yourself with guilt and shame. It also means you have complete authority to eat as much as you want as long as you don't overstuff yourself and eat things that are medically restricted. If you live by this principle, you are going to detach labels from food. They will no longer be good or bad. You also need to realize that no food is going to make you a bad person, unhealthy, addicted or rampant. By doing so, you are letting go of any need for binging or eating emotionally. You understand that all foods are available and up for grabs whenever your body feels. When you try to make peace with your food, you don't just eat everything in one sitting. You see it as a journey of giving up on food rules you have engraved in your mind and unlearning and exploring new foods, what they taste like, and their importance. Here's how you do this.

How to Make Peace with Food?

The first thing you need to do is begin with making a list of all the items you don't like. You can even rate them from somewhat likable to least likable. Once you have a list, pick one item from it and buy it for the sake of trying it. Purchase it in multiple servings so that you are just not eating them because intuitive eating tells you to.

This is a practice that inculcate the message in you that no food is good, bad or off-limits. All foods serve a purpose, including the one you dislike. Be it a pint of ice cream, a bag of chips or broccoli, they all have calories that your body requires to gain energy. Maintaining a balance between the things you like and things you don't will keep your nutritional levels in place and you won't have to make any sacrifices by ditching the things you occasionally eat that are delicious or never eat because they are disgusting!

Next, time your meals. You need to be mindful of whatever you are eating in a place free of distraction. You also don't need to be extra slow or fast like you are in some sort of a rush.

And finally, sit down to finish the meal using all your senses. You may want to journalize all the feelings you have while you eat whether it is pride, guilt or shame.

4. Challenge the Food Police

What is a food policy and how can you challenge it? The food police are all those thoughts that determine what foods you should eat and what foods are bad for you. Sadly, the media has shaped our minds into making that distinction, preventing our internal cues to decide what is best for us. What follows is shame and guilt when we have something from the forbidden food group when it shouldn't be. This food policy is always critiquing us on our choices and making decisions for us. The food police can take the shape of your parents telling you to slim down or no guy will ever find you attractive or a friend who doesn't want you to look fat at her wedding because you are the maid-of-honor. But most of the time, it is our own thoughts that become our biggest enemies and dictate our choices for us.

When we quiet the food police and listen to our internal bias, we allow ourselves a rare opportunity to make good decisions based on things that are pleasurable and satisfying. This is what this principle is all about! Do you want to learn of ways you can challenge the food police? Look below.

How to Challenge the Food Police?

- **Don't make judgments**

Although we have been repeating the mantra of eating whatever you want and whenever you want, this doesn't mean that you have the full liberty to ignore all nutritional values and indulge in foods such as processed meats and fizzy drinks. It is true that you have the freedom to choose, but you are also expected to act mindfully.

So, you start with observation without judgment. Suppose you are consuming protein without any fruits or veggies. You don't need to think constantly that this is bad or judge your food choice. You also don't need to think about how much you will need to run on the treadmill just so you can burn off the calories. You also don't need to make up for the meal you had by having ONLY fruits and veggies at dinner.

What you are doing is judging instead of enjoying and savoring your food. Even if it is an oily steak, it still holds important nutritional value. Even if you are at a dinner party or wedding that has a hearty and calorie-rich menu, you don't need to feel guilty about eating it or not. This principle teaches us that you need to stop judging your food choices, especially when it is your body that is craving for the meal. And you certainly don't need to punish yourself for it later.

- **Don't aim for perfection the first time**

It isn't a movie where the first time you try eating intuitively, you become the best at it. You need to keep practicing over and over again until you get it. Intuitive eating takes time and patience. Since you can't stop eating, don't think of it as a one-time gig that you can gloat about with your friends on your next brunch. Instead, think of it as a lifestyle change and its implications on your life. Besides, you have your whole life to figure out your body's needs. This isn't a race, and no one is chasing after you. So, instead of diving right into it and expecting to come out victorious and a perfectionist, see it as a gradual process with positive results.

If the food police are getting on your nerves just because you had too many donuts last night at your promotion party, remember that not every day will not be like that and it is okay to take out some time to have fun with food. You don't need to beat yourself up because of that and then stay away from donuts for a whole week. A day's eating isn't going to make you fat and it certainly shouldn't demotivate you.

- **Get support from friends to join your team**

Since changing your eating habits will be difficult at the start, how about you get some of your friends to fight off the food police? Since there aren't any hard and fast rules to follow when eating intuitively, having a support group will only make it more fun and less of a regime. Share the ridiculous rules that most diets want you to abide by and talk about the things and actions that lead to self-pity, emotional eating, shame, and guilt concerning food choices.

5. Feel Your Fullness

This step involves complete awareness while you're eating. Once you decide to eat intuitively, you need to get rid of your previous habits around food. For instance, if you just came off a diet or meal plan that you had been practicing for months, you may find it difficult to identify when you are full. Therefore, before we talk about this in detail, understand that it is going to be a process and you will keep learning as you go along. Feeling your fullness isn't about demonizing fullness, but to chart how you feel after the consumption of various foods, and you can keep in mind this question: Are you able to differentiate between the different textures and tastes without judging yourself?. Feeling fullness is also a blessing in disguise as you remind yourself about the availability of food which prevents overeating. This is especially important when coming off a restrictive diet as your chances to go on a binge is at its highest. It is also pivotal to note that it is okay to eat when you are extremely hungry, even if you just had a meal a couple of hours ago. However, you must remember to stop eating before you feel full. This is how you respect your body's cues by not quieting its demands but also not going all in. This balance between the two extremes is what this principle is all about.

Below are some great ways to get you started!

How to Respect Your Fullness?

Before you begin eating, chart how hungry you are. This will help you time your next meal and also allow you to keep track of your fullness when you feel it.

As important it is for you to be physically hungry, it doesn't mean you need to starve yourself before your next meal. If you wait until you are too hungry, you will not be able to track your fullness when you reach it as your mind will still be too tempted by the food that is in front of it. The likelihood of you overeating will increase and it isn't something you want.

The next important thing that you should note is to avoid eating when you are distracted. When you are planning to start eating, ensure that you have switched off your TV, placed aside your phone, and you're not distracted mentally. Did you know that you eat 25% more when you're watching TV? It is also best to minimize the conversations at the dinner table as it will make it harder for you to time and track your fullness.

There shouldn't be any rushing with food. It isn't a race. You don't have to munch everything down before the lunch hour is over. Take your time, slowly biting and savoring each bite. Ideally, you should take out at least 15 to 20 minutes for every meal. Doing so will allow you to take note of your fullness when you reach it and prevent overeating. This is only possible if you listen to your gut-brain carefully and read the cues your body signals.

Use the fullness scale to measure how full you physically feel after a meal. Did you reach complete satisfaction or not? If yes, then by how much?

Next, you need to drop the "clean your plate" mentality. If you feel full when your plate still has food on it, there is no obligation that you must clean it. Listen to your body instead of listening to external pressure. You need to stop when you feel full.

Allow yourself to have some compassion and grace. Since intuitive eating is a gradual process that takes time and practice, forgive yourself if, at some point, you pass comfortable satiety. There will be days when, despite being intuitive eating, you will overeat or feel uncomfortably full. So, don't beat yourself up about it. Intuitive eating is all about forgiving yourself and letting go.

6. Discover the Satisfaction Factor

Discovering your level of satisfaction is all about finding pleasure in eating again. You may be wondering how this principle is any different from the principle #5. Here's how. This principle is about finding the distinction between being full and being satisfied. Has it ever happened to you that despite being super full, you still have cravings for certain foods? Like you want to eat more but your stomach thinks otherwise. If yes, then this is the difference between being full but not satisfied. This also happens when we substitute something for something else. You really wanted to eat a cheeseburger with fries, but you ate a salad instead because your diet tells you to. Do you really think you will be satisfied at all? Yes, you will be full, but not satisfied.

Intuitive eating forbids this. It suggests that you eat the one thing you are craving for instead of those ten other foods you eat because you are bound by some rules. Not only will you feel happier and satisfied, but you will also save yourself from the angst. What you eat shouldn't just be about filling your stomach, it should also fill you with content and joy. The only way you will feel it is if you eat whatever you want. If you need help to better understand whether you are satisfied with what you ate or not, here are a few tips to get you started with.

How to Feel Satisfied After a Meal or Snack?

- **Step 1: Talk to Yourself**

The first step involves asking yourself what you're really craving. Next, sit down and think about this for a minute: what drives most of your food choices? Is it some external pressure or the food police? Then try to recall the last meal where you truly felt like you treated yourself with the best? How long was it? If you can't even recall the last time you had something you really wanted to without following those diet rules, then you don't experience satisfaction often.

Don't make your next meal the same. Think about what you really want to eat right now. Is it grilled cheese, a pizza or a slice of cake? Whatever it is, just remember to stop eating when you're full and aim for a middle spot on your hunger and fullness scale. Satisfaction should be the goal.

- **Step 2: Think About the Food Mindfully**

Once you have sat down for a meal, don't just gobble it up like a robot. Instead, indulge all your senses into it. This will elevate your experience and make you feel better. It's really like foreplay and the anticipation. The more you have it, the better you will feel later.

Think about how it looks, how it smells, and what it tastes like. Is the temperature right? Does its texture excite you? The more explicit and detailed you are about the food, the more satisfied you will be.

- **Step 3: Think of It as an Experience**

Remember, you aren't just eating; you are also enjoying it. How will you be able to enjoy it? When there are zero distractions in your way. Limit the casual chit chat whilst eating: find an ergonomic chair to sit down and eat, get all your required cutlery in front of your beforehand, have a glass of water beside you, and set aside any gadget that might distract you with a pop-up message. The goal is to allow yourself to tune in with your body and go on an exciting journey together. Savor every bite and notice all those feelings that arise within you every time you take another bite. You must also cut down any judgments that keep humming into your ears that what you are eating is going to make you fat.

- **Step 4: Check-in with Yourself**

Lastly, do check in with yourself. An ideal time to eat and enjoy food is when you are mildly hungry. When you are starving to death, your first instinct is to chomp down as fast as you can. If you aren't hungry at all and eating for the sake of eating only, you won't be able to enjoy it. If, at any point you realize that the food you are eating doesn't excite you anymore, stop. This is what the originators of the intuitive program call the last bite threshold. When you reach the last bite threshold, even the most exciting of foods become your "normal" and you no longer enjoy it. Therefore, stopping at that point is a must. Besides, you can always have more of it when the craving arises again.

7. Honor Your Feelings

Although eating for emotional reasons is looked down upon in most diets, there is something remarkable about it too. When you eat to cope with stress or emotions, at least you acknowledge that there is something wrong and needs attention. Instead of eating, you can sit down and think about those feelings and try to resolve those problems that trigger emotional eating in the first place. Moreover, you can even look at other ways to cope with your feelings as the emotional eating is often accompanied by shame and guilt later. So, if you want to save yourself from all that, consider this a heads up. The next time you feel sad, stressed or just down for no reason, don't think of food as your savior. It may make you feel better for some time, but it does have some unlikeable consequences. So, leave that bottle of wine for a happier occasion because if you don't, you are going to wake up with a massive hangover that will make you hate yourself even more than the previous night.

How to Cope Without Food?

If you are looking for some other ways to cope with your feelings, here are some great tips to get you by.

- **Seek Nurturing**

Tribole and Resch suggest that to cope with your emotions, it is best to seek nurture from something other than food. When you are occupied with other means of nurturing, the thought of eating loses its appeal as your needs are met. Think of food as a part of the healing process but not the default answer for everything. All you need is some encouragement and nourishment which can easily come from:

1. Taking a nap to forget about the problem
2. Listening to some relaxing tunes to distract your mind
3. Taking a long shower to treat yourself
4. Meditation to really think about the problems, their root cause, and possible solutions
5. Getting a spa facial, massage, or manicure and pedicure

- **Acknowledge Your Troubles**

You need to acknowledge the things that are troubling you. Will they go away without bringing food into it? Sometimes it is okay to not feel okay. You can always pick up the phone and dial a friend's number and ask them to come over. Or you can confront the issue or the person that is making you feel that way. You mustn't always think of food as your go-to medication.

- **Distract Yourself**

If you still don't feel better after a consultation or confrontation, try moving away from it by tricking your mind into doing something else. If you think that you might not be able to resist eating, the best way is to remove yourself from the place where you have easy access to it. For example, if you are at home feeling low and you know there is food in the kitchen. What do you? Go for a walk or on a drive. Or pick up a book or get cleaning. Distractions not only take your mind off your troubles; they often serve as a means to reduce the intensity of it. An hour ago, you might have felt like crying your eyes out, but now after Marie Kondo-ing your room, you might not feel that way. The feelings of sadness will still be there but less intense. The less intense your feelings, the less likely you are to go near food for comfort.

8. Respect Your Body

Although body love is equally important to practice, this principle is more about the liberation of the body rather than self-love. This is about you accepting the way you look, your height and weight and features. It is about acknowledging the fact that we were all made different and regardless of trying hard to look like someone else, say your sibling, your neighbor or a model on the cover of Vogue, we need to seek acceptance about the way we look. Of course, there isn't any harm trying to look better, but not at the stake of your mental and physical health. Therefore, wishing that you were a different height or shape means you don't respect your body the way that it is. This principle is also about ditching the fatphobia culture in society and aims to see everyone as they are without the weight stigmas. If you don't respect the body you have and continuously feel like some diet, supplement or physical activity is going to change it, then it will be difficult for you to practice intuitive eating as you will be constantly worrying about weight loss and your overall appearance.

How to Respect Your Body?

- **Keep It Hydrated**

Drinking more water should be your primary goal. A hydrated body is full of energy. The skin feels better, the organs function smoothly, and it makes you feel less hungry all the time. This is one of the most important ways to honor your body to prevent any digestive and kidney-related conditions.

- **Get Enough Sleep**

Standardly, your body needs at least 5 to 7 hours of sleep every night. A lot of times, we compromise our sleep for things like workout, work, and household chores. However, a lack of sleep has its side effects as well and they take no time to show in a fatigued, sluggish and cranky you. Besides, what's the point of a workout if you aren't allowing your body enough rest to recharge itself for another day? Thus, the second most important way to honor your body is to get a good night's sleep. If you suffer from a sleep disorder, do try taking short naps in the afternoon to cover up for the sleep lost at night. A good night's sleep does wonders for your body, mind, and skin, so try to honor your body with it.

- **Appreciate Your Body**

Next, you mustn't forget to appreciate what your body does for you from carrying your weight to functioning properly to make you feel like "you" every day. Think about it, if it wasn't fit or weak, would you have been able to accomplish all that you can?

- **Limit the "Fat" Talk**

Limit the negative talk about the way you look. We all talk bad about our bodies. Some of us want to have a bigger chest, while others want their thighs to look thinner. No good has ever come from talking about your flaws unless you are willing to make a change for it. Besides, even with all those flaws, your body doesn't let you down, so why do you?

- **Go Shopping**

Since it is all about honoring your body, how can we not mention clothes? Honoring your body also includes dressing it in the right, well-fitted clothes. We have to find a balance between too fitted or too loose. Basically, wear what looks good and compliments your body without making it compromise. Dress comfortably, so that you allow some room for your body to breathe freely.

9. Exercise: Feel the Difference

There is no compulsion for you to hit the gym every day when adopting an intuitive approach. However, a sedentary lifestyle isn't encouraged either. Keep your body moving so that it doesn't develop a sluggish or hunched posture with time. If you do opt for some physical exercises, opt for the ones that are sustainable and enjoyable. Don't waste your time trying to do exercises solely for burning fat or losing weight. instead, pick something you enjoy or else you won't be able to do it for long.

How to Become an Intuitive Exerciser?

To get you started, here are a few tips:

1. Respect the needs of your body and listen to the internal cues and triggers. For instance, if running on the treadmill causes chest pains, don't continue with it. Chest pain is a clear indication that your body isn't ready for running.
2. Think of fatigue as a cue as well. If some strenuous high-intensity interval training (HIIT) is leaving you with zero energy levels throughout the day, then maybe you need to tone it down and try something less intensive and hardcore to build your stamina first.

3. Next, you need to have a purpose for exercising. Why are you doing it? Is it to lose weight, burn calories or simply stay active and healthy? The more convincing your reason, the likelier you are to continue with it.
4. Expand your options when it comes to exercises. Don't just go for a jog or work on your upper body area only, aim for a variety of exercises so you continue to enjoy the mix and don't think of it as a workout. For instance, if you are into sports like tennis, boxing or cricket, these can be exercises as they keep you on your toes and include movement. So, if you aren't the gym-type, try taking up a sport you enjoy and consider it as your physical activity.

10. Honor Your Health with Gentle Nutrition

Although, the very approach of intuitive eating encourages us to eat whatever we feel like, it doesn't mean that you can put everything in your body. Oxymoron, right? Well, the researchers Tibole and Resch wanted the practitioners of intuitive eating lifestyle to suggest that whenever we feel like eating anything, they must evaluate the nutritional value of it. Good nutrition must still be one's top priority. You must make food choices that are healthy in general and honor your health. Thus, think about incorporating more fruits and vegetables or try having them as a side dish to some protein or carb-dense food. Trying this approach won't make you completely get rid of food that you really wish to enjoy, but it also has some nutritional value to balance out the unhealthy fats.

How to Honor Your Food with Gentle Nutrition?

What does honoring your food with gentle nutrition actually mean and how do you do it? Think of this as an amalgamation of all the principles we previously covered.

This last principle is all about expanding your options by giving your body the choice to choose from a variety of foods with good nutritional values. Indulge in foods that make you feel good without any judgments but are also good for your body. It is also about becoming more aware of your body's needs. Honoring your food also means that you listen to your body's reaction to all the foods you eat. Learn how it reacts. When your stomach hurts that means that the food you consumed didn't sit well with your body, thus, you might want to hold back on that particular food. Similarly, if after the consumption of a certain food, and you feel not only do you feel happy but also more energized and focused, then you might make this food a staple to your meal.

Next, you need to find a balance between not eating enough and not eating too much.

Keep in mind that there are no forbidden foods anymore. You can have all that your body craves without feeling guilty or trying to substitute it for something much healthier. Every food has some nutritional value, so don't try to always aim for those that rank highest on the nutrition chart and be full but not satisfied.

And lastly, don't be too hard on yourself. There will be days and events where you eat more than you should have, but that doesn't mean that you need to go on a diet for the rest of the week to balance out the extra calories. It is okay to have some less than stellar days. No one is judging you except yourself. Sometimes, it is okay to not be a rude critic and let go.

Take Away

This chapter takes a detailed look at each of the 10 principles of intuitive eating that serves as the basis of the overall approach to eating. From honoring your hunger, fullness, and body, it also covers aspects like the importance of good nutrition, the role of physical activity, how one can get started with intuitive eating, coping with emotions other than with food, and how to quiet the food police and so much more. This chapter not only describes each principle in its core essence but also teaches how they can be implemented in daily life, so you can reap the best results.

Chapter 4: Intuitive Eating Struggles

A dieter may say that a diet is a solution to all your problems, but an intuitive eater will tell you that all the answers you seek are within yourself. It is true, all the answers we seek are within us because it was designed by Mother nature that way.

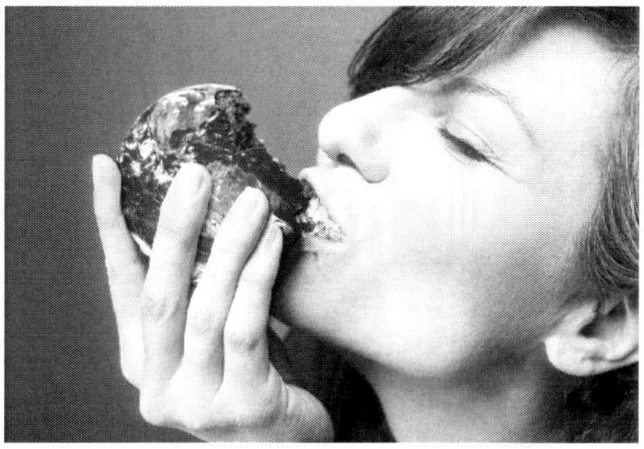

Call it a Buddha approach, but this is exactly what intuitive eating teaches us. The idea behind intuitive eating is to reconnect with our inner self, tune into it to let us guide ourselves with its wisdom and help us figure out a way to eat the right way.

Unlike traditional diets, intuitive eating allows its followers some wiggle room to interpret their body needs and execute them. This is what makes it such an ideal approach to eating. There are no limitations or bindings. However, it is the same flexibility that makes it so easy to give up on intuitive eating as most people consider it a failure as it doesn't make them lose weight. But it was never the actual goal of eating intuitively. Many people see it as unrealistic because there aren't any restrictions, which they consider a requisite to any diet form.

In this chapter, we are going to be looking at some of the most concerning myths, and mistakes that people make when it comes to intuitive eating and hopefully change the views of those who regard it as a failure or unrealistic.

7 Myths and Misconceptions About Intuitive Eating

Myth #1: Eating Like Children = Eating Junk Food

Just because intuitive eating permits that we pay heed to our cravings, it doesn't necessarily mean that we will only crave junk food. The premise of eating intuitively is to go back to how you were supposed to eat, just like a child does. People often mistake it for only junk food. Ask yourself ladies, has your child ever showed interest in some vegetable or fruit? Do they always want a French fry or sweets? Yes, they may want more of them but not always.

When intuitive eating tells you to eat like kids, it mostly means to eat only when you are hungry and stop when you are full — just like kids do!

Myth #2: There Is No Structure with Intuitive Eating

Again, this is just a myth. Intuitive eating has the most flexible structure if you are interested to know as it allows each follower to tailor the principles as they see fit and as per their individual needs. There is no one way to eat or drink, there isn't a set time when you should eat, and there aren't any restrictions either.

True, there aren't any hard and fast rules like nearly all diets have, but isn't that what makes it unique and adaptable? If someone needs some guidance, they have the 10 principles to get started. Once you work your way around them and follow them passionately, then there comes a time when you no longer need to abide by any rules and regulations and eat whenever you want.

It can be slightly challenging to adopt at first, especially for someone who has a history of yo-yo dieting, but it's not impossible.

Myth #3: It's Much Easier Than Dieting

Wrong, it is much harder to adopt. Why? Because unlike most diets that come with a given set of rules and regulations that the follower must abide by throughout the designated period, intuitive eating comes with no such pamphlet of instructions. It is challenging because it rejects the diet mentality — something we are so used to for ages. There isn't any prize associated with it either. It involves changing your old food habits and adopting new ones. It is about changing your attitude towards food which is difficult. Laid out rules are much easier to follow through as they promise some benefit or prize in the end.

Myth #4: It Is for People with an Eating Disorder

It is for everyone wishing to eat healthier, beat cravings, and set themselves free from the shackles of fad diets. It especially works wonders for those coming off of an eating disorder as they usually have a difficult relationship with food. Intuitive eating is all about mending that relationship and help the survivors get back on their feet and eat healthily.

Many people also think that intuitive eating isn't for people with eating disorders. Although, it is true that when people suffer from some health condition or disorder, their hunger and fullness scale isn't accurate or perceivable. There are days where they may feel hungry all day and then days where they can go for 12+ hours without food.

Even then, it doesn't mean that intuitive eating isn't ideal for them. Intuitive eating is more than just living by the hunger and fullness scale. There are many other principles of intuitive eating that can be adopted such as exercising, making peace with food, honoring the body, respecting its needs, and not giving in to the temptations of emotional eating.

Myth #5: Intuitive Eating Isn't for You If You Have Dietary Restrictions

Thinking that you won't be able to adopt the intuitive eating approach if you have dietary restrictions is another common myth amongst newbies. In fact, it is also one of the most commonly asked FAQ on many online forums and discussions. If someone suffers from a dietary restriction, say lactose intolerance, then they must ensure that their eating intuitively doesn't come in the way of the restrictions. Yes, they will have to honor their body by giving up things with lactose, but it doesn't mean they can't practice all the principles of intuitive eating. They just have been cautious of their cravings and ensure they don't cause any disrespect to their bodies by eating something that is not good for their body.

Myth #6: You Have to Give in to Every Craving That Comes Along

It may seem like it does promote eating whatever you want and whenever you want, but it also promotes eating things that honor your body. How can one honor their bodies? By choosing things that are healthier and more fulfilling with nutritional value. When people begin eating intuitively, they begin to realize that their cravings go away after a while. This happens because they never starved their body when a craving arose and ate whatever it craved. When you stop limiting yourself from something, the urge to have it diminishes as well. It's a lot like when you want that scarf from the jewelry shop that is out of stock. You keep refreshing the website every few days to check if it is back in stock. And then one day when it finally is, you buy it. Then you wear it enthusiastically for a few weeks or months and then it just becomes another staple in your closet that you will soon forget about.

Cravings work in the same way. They hold their charm as long as they are restricted. Intuitive eating is more about deciding what your body needs rather than controlling your food choices. Besides, if you practice intuitive eating or are in the process of becoming one, you honor your body and its needs. At the same time, you also begin to make sound judgments about your food choices. Instead of simply giving in, you understand why you have that desire and where is it coming from. Is an emotional setting driving it or is it more of physiological hunger?

Myth #7: You Are Eating Intuitively Because You Have Given Up

If you think that someone around you has opted for intuitive eating is because nothing else seemed to work, then you are absolutely wrong. Yes, they may have given up, but not on themselves, but on the diet culture that pressurized them to continue with fad and unhealthy diets so they can look like those cover girls. They gave up on the culture that kept telling them that they were somehow flawed and not good enough. If that is the case, then a good thing that they gave up. They are now on the route to physical and emotional happiness.

7 Mistakes You Are Making with Intuitive Eating

Did you know, the number one reason that all these misconceptions and myths form is because we make multiple mistakes with intuitive eating? As long as we don't understand the core concept, we will fail to practice and incorporate it into our daily lives and become an intuitive eater like we were when we were kids. Therefore, to put the above myths to rest, it is pivotal that we take a look at all the mistakes we make while trying to eat intuitively to be able to practice it better.

Mistake #1: Thinking You Can Eat Whatever You Want Whenever You Want

Yes, intuitive eating allows you to pick whichever food your body craves and wishes to eat, but it also reminds us to treat our body with honor and respect. How do you do that? By ensuring that you feed it with good nutrition. Now, if you are following the diet to the tee, you will stop craving junk food as you realize that it leaves you feeling lethargic and sluggish. You want to feel energetic, satisfied, and fulfilled which can only come from healthy eating and limiting the greasy, fatty, and "fast" food along the way.

Mistake #2: Not Giving Up the Diet Mentality

How many times will we have to remind you that intuitive eating isn't a diet? One of the primary reasons people give up on intuitive eating is because they see it as a means to lose weight. Yes, it helps in doing so but it was never its core intention. The core intention was to get in touch with our inner selves and let it take control of our eating choices and habits. If you didn't come with this intention in mind, then perhaps, it is true that it won't work for you.

You need to give up on the diet mentality, which also happens to be the first principle of intuitive eating. The more you cling to it, the lesser your chances of becoming an intuitive eater. You need to trust your body and let it guide you. You need to appreciate the way it looks rather than trying to change it with poor dietary choices that lead to health conditions and hormonal imbalances.

Yes, it may seem difficult to not think about the diet mentality or let it go, but you must if you wish to become an intuitive eater.

Mistake #3: Believing You Can't Lose Weight with Intuitive Eating

There is tons of research, later discussed in chapter 10 of the book, which proposes how remarkable it can be to help you lose weight. If you recently just came off a diet, your biggest worry right now must be if you will continue to lose weight or worse, will you regain all your lost weight. Here's the thing with intuitive eating, if you pay attention to your body's needs and only eat when you're moderately hungry and stop when you're moderately full, you will see the pointer on your weighing scale fall back. Moreover, since there will be no restrictions as to what you can eat, there will rarely be any cravings. If you continue down this road, you will also begin to notice that your body will stop craving for fun foods as it was naturally designed to function on fruits, veggies, nuts, and other nutritious foods.

All these aspects of intuitive eating make for a classic weight-loss recipe, doesn't it? So how can you not lose weight with it?

Mistake #4: Continuing with Food Restrictions

When eating intelligently, there are no restrictions on what you are eating and in what quantity as long as you eat when you're hungry and stop when you're full. There are no rules with intuitive eating which means you can quiet the food police that tell you what to eat and what not to eat. Try to eat more of the foods that pass the health test and are loaded with nutrients like vitamin, iron, Omega-3, and good carbs.

Besides, when you stop denying your body certain foods, it will also put an end to your cravings which often result in binge or emotional eating.

Mistake #5: You Disregard Physical Activity

Just because you are no longer keeping a check of calories with every meal doesn't give you the right to become a couch potato and give up exercising. Staying active is a crucial part of intuitive eating. You need to burn what you are eating and that means sweating up or making your heart race faster for at least 30 minutes per day. It doesn't have to be a hardcore, rigorous fitness regime, but definitely something that gets your blood gushing through your veins faster.

Start with something you enjoy doing, say walking and then pace it up to brisk walking and later full-on jogging to build your stamina and improve your digestion and metabolic rate.

Mistake #6: Thinking It's About Failing or Succeeding

There is no concept of failure or success in intuitive eating. It isn't a race but rather a process that takes time and practice to learn and live by. Despite this, most people just assume that since they aren't losing weight, the diet is a failure and move onto another one. If you keep thinking this way about intuitive eating and stay focused on just the results, you will always be judging and critiquing your choices.

Intuitive eating isn't about perfectionism but rather continuing to progress towards a healthier lifestyle. So don't be too critical of yourself and don't stand on the weighing scale every single day hoping for a miracle. The miracle is learning to listen to your internal messages.

Mistake #7: You Think You Have a Free Hand with Portions

Portion control may not be the core concept of intuitive eating, but there is a strong emphasis on stopping when you're full which is almost the same thing. Since intuitive eating isn't a "diet," many people believe there aren't any restrictions when it comes to portions. True, you can eat whatever you want but in a considerate amount. Though, don't go measuring how many bites you have taken. Listen to the inner cues that tell you when to stop. With time, you will notice how good you become at controlling your portions and stopping when you are no longer hungry.

Take Away

In this chapter, we take a look at the various myths that revolve around intuitive eating and set the score right. Next, we looked at the many mistakes intuitive eaters make when their just starting out. this consists of things like not knowing when to stop, thinking it is only about eating, not honoring your body with the right nutrition, and underestimating the importance of exercise.

Chapter 5: Intuitive Eating and Common Eating Disorders

Eating disorders are a combination of illnesses that include irregular eating habits, posing a serious concern about your weight and shape. Disturbances in eating with either excessive or inadequate intake of food are what lead to a disorder. Eating disorders can develop at any age and both men and women are equally at risk. Eating disorders are most common among teenagers and adults, mostly developed due to social media or psychological pressure from society. There are a number of medical, therapeutic, and nutritional treatments to stop and recover from eating disorders, intuitive eating being one of them. In this chapter, not only will we take a look at some of the most common eating disorders but also learn how intuitive eating as a treatment can help recover from them. The reason eating disorders need to be addressed is because they usually coexist with multiple other health conditions like substance abuse, anxiety or depression. Therefore, recovery from an eating disorder is the first step to treating other crucial disorders like depression and substance abuse.

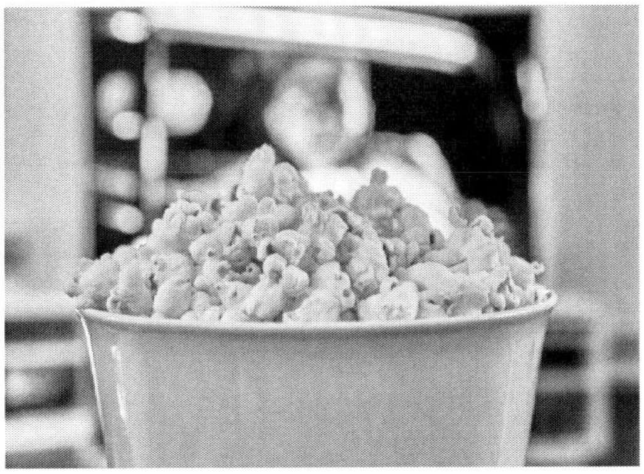

Anorexia Nervosa

This is commonly known as anorexia, and it is an eating disorder that involves an abnormally low body weight. If you know of someone suffering from anorexia or are anorexic yourself, your biggest fear and concern is gaining weight. You have a distorted weight perception and have been eating restrictively for months or years. You indulge in extreme efforts to continue looking for a certain shape and having a certain weight. You have given up on carbs completely, exercise excessively, are misusing diet aids, laxatives, enemas and vomit your food after consumption. Although you already have a significantly low body weight, you still live in the fear of gaining weight and never stop and accept the way you are.

Causes

There isn't just a single explanation of what causes anorexia. It is a complex lifestyle and arises from a multitude of emotional, social, and biological factors. Perhaps, the most prominent cause is our infatuation with thinness today. Ever seen Victoria's Secret models? As much as you adore their figure, it isn't ideal. In France, they have put a ban on models walking the ramp that are too thin as it gives other women unrealistic expectations about how they should look. Some other factors that contribute to developing this eating disorder include:

- Perfectionism
- Low self-esteem
- Body dissatisfaction
- Emotional difficulties
- Strict dieting
- History of physical or emotional abuse
- Troubled past

Symptoms

How do you know if someone is anorexic or in the process of becoming one? There are several signs and symptoms they depict commonly. These include:

- Restrictive eating
- Being underweight or rapidly losing significant weight over a short amount of time
- Obsessing about calories in foods
- Being ritualistic with food such as hiding it, cutting it into short pieces or avoiding to eat in a social gathering
- A continued fixation about recipes, cooking, and food in general
- Depression
- Thinning or loss of hair
- Amenorrhea
- Feeling cold
- Development of tiny hairs on face and body
- Preferring isolation and withdrawal from family and friends

Where Intuitive Eating Comes In?

Since it is a serious condition, medical treatments and therapy have proven most effective as recovery methods. However, since the obsession with food restrictions, calories counting, and weight loss is concerning, an intuitive eating regime can also help in the process of recovery. Since intuitive eating encourages eating when one feels like it, doesn't forbid any foods and promotes a healthy weight and shape by listening to internal cues, it can greatly help the patient recover and restore a healthy body weight by implementing the principles of the intuitive eating program.

Bulimia Nervosa

Bulimia nervosa is another concerning the type of eating disorder in which the individual suffers from a mental illness characterized by repeated binging and purging episodes. In the simplest of terms, think of it as a really bad on and off relationship with food. The individual doesn't know when to stop eating and continues to eat despite being full. Women with bulimia often have a hard time channeling their food-related urges elsewhere and always look to food when they are emotionally or mentally unstable.

Causes

Although the exact cause is still unknown to medical experts, countless research and patient history deduce that one's personality traits, eating patterns, and thinking have a crucial role to play. There are also some environmental or biological factors involved. Like anorexia, it also starts with one's dissatisfaction towards their body. Bulimics are extremely concerned about the way they look, and their body appears. It is also common to notice that those who suffer from bulimia nervosa have poor self-worth and the fear of gaining weight never leaves their minds.

Symptoms

Someone suffering from bulimia nervosa depicts a number of unique signs and symptoms. These include:

- Weight fluctuations
- Damaged blood vessels under the eyes
- Electrolyte imbalances
- Enlarged glands under the jawline and in the neck
- Oral trauma
- Chronic gastric reflux
- Inflammation of the esophagus
- Chronic dehydration
- Infertility

Where Intuitive Eating Comes In?

When recovering from bulimia, patients are encouraged to see intuitive eating as a healthy habit to adopt. It is prescribed so that the individual is able to reestablish a healthy relationship with food, their mind, and body. However, learning to eat intuitively for any bulimic patient is both difficult and stressful. They can't adhere to the 10 principles if they continue to depict the behaviors associated with bulimia. Since the patient had been binge eating for long, it will be difficult to understand hunger cues and prevent eating mindlessly every few hours. They will also need to track their need for food and cater to any digestive issues that arise with the withdrawal of the old habit.

Since the individual will have a tough time regulating their hunger and stopping when they're full, it is best to seek professional help of a dietician or nutritionist to help them get started with foods they can eat and foods they need to stop binging on. Only when the repeated behavior of eating stops, can bulimia be treated.

Avoidant Restrictive Food Intake Disorder (ARFID)

It is an eating disorder characterized by a continuous failure to meet standard nutritional or energy levels which leads to one or more of the following issues.

- Significant weight loss
- Significant nutritional deficiency
- External feeding or dependence on oral nutrition
- An interference in psychological functioning

Causes

Like most eating disorders, there isn't just one culprit to place blame on. Although evolving studies have suggested that disordered eating breeds from multifaceted chemistry of sociocultural, genetic, and psychological factors.

Symptoms

Some of the most prominent signs and symptoms observed in someone living with AFRID includes:

- A limited list of eat-able foods
- Choosing to eat foods with similar characteristics such as colorless or crunchy
- Avoiding fruits, vegetables, and proteins
- Elimination of certain food and vowing to never eat them again
- Strict preferences on how their food is prepared
- Skipping entire food groups
- Food limitations which affect their social behaviors
- Demonstrating stress and anxiety when presented with something other than their preferred food
- Multiple nutrient deficiencies
- Poor weight gain

Where Intuitive Eating Comes In?

Changes are conceivable for people suffering from ARFID. Once intuitive eating is adopted as a means of treatment, it will help the patient with relying on internal cues in contrast to oral and external cues of hunger. Then it will also help in providing the patient with an abundance of nutrients in various forms such as raw fruits and vegetables, juices and dairy. This will also prevent significant weight loss which can lead to anorexia nervosa.

Binge Eating

We already understand what binge eating is all about as it has been discussed several times in the book earlier, however, since it is also an eating disorder, and fairly a common one these days with the whole Netflix and chill theme, it is crucial that we understand the long-term effects it can have on our digestion, metabolism, and overall health. Not only will the unusually large consumption of usually fun foods add to your weight, the amount of carbs and cholesterol in them also slows down heart rate, making one feel less active and lethargic throughout the day. Going on a binge is also linked to a bloated tummy and gassy stomach and an increased risk of gastric reflux, which is both painful and uncomfortable.

Of course, there will be some occasions when you can eat as much as you want and have as many meals you desire, but don't let it become a habit. A lot of people have trouble eating normally after the holidays when they have down some hearty eating. No wonder, so many people's New Year resolutions involve getting in shape and thus gyms and sports clubs get so many new clients in the first week of January. Besides, there is a limit to overeating, and the sooner you realize that it is getting out of control, the easier it will be for you to bounce back to your routine eating habits.

Causes

There are a number of contributing factors that make one want to binge eat and develop an eating disorder. These factors include:

Psychological Factors: Psychological factors such as depression, stress, and anxiety have been linked with binge eating. Those who happen to binge eat also have a difficult time coping with their emotions and feelings and thus eat as a way to deal with them. They also tend to suffer from low-self-esteem and dissatisfaction with the way they look.

Biological Factors: Binge eating may also be a result due to hormonal imbalances in your body. Have you changed your diet, your sleeping habits or your workout routine? All these can lead to hormonal imbalances and irregularities. It can also be genetic. If your family has this habit of consuming food whenever they can get their hands on it despite being full, then maybe you have developed it because of that too. Food addictions also run in some families where the mother or the father is obsessive about eating something particular and the child becomes an addict too.

Cultural and social factors: Traumatic experiences can also cause binge eating. For centuries, food has been a staple for comfort for humans. They eat when they are stressed so they distract themselves. Sexual abuse, history of torn family relationships or a bad breakup can all increase one's chances of turning to food for comfort. Social pressure also has a certain role to make one binge eat. The constant pressure from your family, friends, and peers to be a certain weight, shape, and height can be too much for someone and make them vulnerable and unable to stop eating.

Symptoms

Although being obese or overweight is linked to unhealthy food habits, it is a telltale sign that one eats past their fullness or binge eat. But can only obese people develop this disorder? Sadly, no. We all are at risk of developing it if we continue to eat despite being full and satiated. If you think you have been eating more than usual, then you might want to check out these symptoms below and hope that you don't have to nod to most or all of them. These include:

- Consuming large quantities of food over a short period of time, say every two or three hours
- Acknowledging that your hunger isn't controllable
- Eating when not hungry or past fullness
- Chomping down food rapidly without worrying about the consequences
- Going on diets every few weeks but with little success
- Feelings of disgust, guilt, shame, and depression about your eating habits
- Eating until uncomfortably full
- Eating alone or in secret

Where Intuitive Eating Comes In?

At its very core, binge eating stems from a biological reaction caused by deprivation around food. It involves responses like eating because you haven't had a certain thing in three weeks and when you finally get your hands on it, it is impossible to stop. So, we can understand it as a reaction to cravings, which intuitive eating can help overcome. Another response to binge eating is something like this: "Oh well, haven't I already screwed up enough? Look at my weight, another slice of cake can't hurt me more." This roots from the fact that one has lost hope in getting into a better and healthy shape with eating right. People who binge eat start believing that there is no going back to what they used to look like. This happens because they have already tried several diets that failed them, and they put on the lost weight sooner than they had anticipated.

Luckily, all these problems have been looked into by the originators of the intuitive eating plan. Dieticians, Tibole and Resch understand these responses very well and thus laid the 10 principles which cater to each of these problems individually. If the binge-eating craze is due to unmet cravings, then intuitive eating encourages to fulfill them, if it is due to lowself-esteem, then intuitive eating also suggests that the moment you start respecting your hunger and your body needs, you will see a significant difference in the way you feel, and when you finally start watching your weight going down on the scale, you will regain your self-esteem and confidence back.

Once restrictions over food have been dealt with, the rest of the problems will dissolve themselves.

Emotional Eating

Emotional eating is eating because you feel emotionally unstable. It usually is a reaction to dissatisfactory emotions like sadness, loneliness, depression or stress. Think of it as a means to suppress negative emotions and feel a little better about your situation. Although there isn't any harm to eat to fill a hole in your heart or to comfort yourself, doing so frequently can become a disorder and a bad one.

Causes

Emotions play a key role in how our body feels. When we feel low, so does our body. When we feel stressed, the body releases the stress hormone cortisol which only worsens the situation we are in. When we feel sad or depressed, it too has a negative impact on our body. So, to uplift one's mood and bring out some positively the brain triggers the craving for something comforting. Unfortunately, whenever we think about comfort, our first choice is food. Maybe it is because it is so readily available and requires little to no movement. And since the body is already feeling down, it doesn't mind either.

Symptoms

Although emotional eaters will let you know that they ate a whole cake or a bag of chips because they felt low or wanted to cry, below are some of the symptoms they also portray. These include:

- Bloated tummy
- Stomachache
- Weight gain
- Eating in secret
- Buying in bulk quantities
- Depression
- Worry
- Shame
- Anxiety
- Isolation and social withdrawal
- Poor skin
- Feel like giving up on everything
- Troubled sleep
- Fatigue and tiredness

Where Intuitive Eating Comes in?

If we go back to the seventh principle of intuitive eating, we understand how emotional eating can be controlled. The principle teaches us to respect our feelings and promotes eating only when one feels hungry. If only we abide by that one principle, emotional eating will be put to an end as you will realize that food isn't the answer to your problems and too much of it can lead to uncomfortable feelings such as gas, bloating, and even fatigue. The moment one realizes that these feelings arise because of eating inappropriately or in large quantities, there is a chance that they would like to give up and eat right.

Next, we also have a principle that teaches us to respect our bodies and honor our hunger. Abiding by them can also help those with emotional eating disorders.

Nighttime Eating Syndrome

It is ironic that despite being a completely different eating disorder from binge eating, all the midnight snackers are also binge eaters. The only difference between the two disorders is that in binge eating, one consumes large quantities of food at short intervals. The nighttime eating syndrome doesn't necessarily involve too much food consumption. It is concerned with the urge to eat in the middle of the night. There are many reasons why snacking after midnight isn't healthy. For starters, those who have the habit of getting up in the night and looking for food in the fridge have interrupted their sleep. Their brain doesn't get enough time to relax and recharge. They also report having difficulty in falling asleep after snacking. Our bodies are designed to begin the process of digestion and metabolism as soon as we take the first bite of our food. Secondly, we have always been advised to have the last meal of our day 2 to 3 hours before bedtime. If we think about it, we are depriving our bodies of both these and eating without being hungry or giving the body time to digest and metabolize. This also adds to our weight and one important reason why people who eat in the middle of the night are obese or overweight.

Causes

Researchers are still deliberating over what causes people to develop this disorder but there hasn't been much research-based evidence yet. Some contributing factors that play an imperative role include hormonal imbalances. When one suffers from a hormonal imbalance, their body doesn't fully function like it is supposed to be. Therefore, the cues of hunger and fullness are often messed up.

Another factor is the habit to have dinner late at night after staying up past midnight. This is quite common among college and high school students as they tend to spend nights studying and binge-eating on whatever is available. Since they are distracted, they often overeat and thus develop it as a habit.

On and off dieting is also responsible for the nighttime eating syndrome. Since dieters avoid eating much throughout the day, when night comes, their body feels deprived of nutrients and thus begin to crave for food. Sometimes the craving is so bad that it can wake you up in the middle of the night due to extreme hunger. The restriction to eat less in the daytime comes out as frustration and hunger at night. And when the snacking continues, it is very seldom that one loses weight and thus becomes even more disappointed and continue to binge eat.

Symptoms

Some of the most common symptoms observed in someone with the nighttime syndrome include:

- Evening hyperphagia
- Morning Anorexia
- Difficulty in falling asleep
- Difficulty in staying asleep
- Experience irritation, anxiety, depression, and agitation which worsens at night.

Where Intuitive Eating Comes In?

Since intuitive eating disregards the diet mentality and instead, promote eating what the body wants, sufferers of the nighttime eating syndrome can adopt the habit of eating everything when the body really wants it. It doesn't have to be tied with time. When body cues are given importance, one learns how to handle their hunger in a timely manner. So when you feel fed and satisfied throughout the day, you won't be craving to snack during the night. Another way intuitive eating may help is to reject timely constraints that one has to eat at a certain time only. Eating in reasonable quantities when hunger strikes can help with the elimination of the need to eat during the night.

How to Eat Intuitively with Dietary Restrictions?

What about people with food intolerances and allergies? Is intuitive eating not for them? Catering to intolerances and allergies are becoming one of the top priorities of many food giants and restaurants. Many even go as far as developing a special separate menu to cater to just those with intolerances and allergies, which is great! But does that mean those with intolerances can't practice eating intuitively? Certainly not!

Here's how someone with, say a lactose intolerance or peanut allergies can continue with the intuitive eating approach and lead a healthy lifestyle.

Recognize Your Limitations

The first step to any disease, be it mental or physical is to accept that you have it and then move onto working towards the other courses of prescribed treatments. The same is the case with people with food restrictions and allergies. The first step is to recognize that you have an intolerance or allergy you have to be cautious about, no matter how frustrating it gets. But don't let that define all your food choices and you certainly don't have to be scared around your food either. Of course, you will have to work with them, but don't let them define you. There is still a lot that you can eat and enjoy to the fullest.

Focus on What You Can Eat

If you have an intolerance or allergy, only certain foods must be restricted. Now, you have two options here. Either you can continue harping that you have an allergy or deal with it and focus on the things you can eat. There is a wide spectrum of food groups and subgroups that you can enjoy. Why worry about that one thing you can't have and lose focus from the things you can have? If you still wish to, you can mourn the elimination of specific foods, but only for some time. When you are done, take a pen and paper and list down all the foods you can eat. We bet you will need more than just a paper or notebook to all the wonderful things you are allowed to eat without worrying about worsening your condition or having an allergic reaction. Once you have a list, notice how many foods you never tried or eat less of.

Satisfy Your Cravings

We all give in to our cravings at times. But what if the food you are craving is restricted? How do you go satisfying that when practicing intuitive eating which urges its followers to eat whatever they feel like and give in to the body cravings? Picture this, the person sitting next to you is enjoying a bowl of homemade pasta and all you can think about is diving right into it. But you are also gluten-intolerant which means it's a big no for you. How will you stop yourself and resist the temptation?

Here's how. Look for some substitute that is equally satisfying. Remember, if intuitive eating is about giving in to your cravings, it is also about eating healthy and feeling good about what you are having. Therefore, look for some substitute that brings out similar feelings from within like that bowl of pasta. It could be some fruits, nuts, a whole-grain item or something similar that you are tempted and excited to eat whenever you get the chance. It may or may not have the same effect on you, but you surely feel much better and satisfied after you eat it.

Focus on How the Food Makes You Feel

An important aspect of the intuitive eating program is how the food makes you feel when you eat it. The goal should be sheer enjoyment, joy, and satisfaction. There are many foods that can make you feel like a million bucks and those are the ones you need to focus more on. Whenever a temptation to have them arises, you don't have to resist it because intuitive eating teaches us so. Focus on how food makes you feel. Does it uplift your mood like ice-cream does for a kid or does it make you feel bloated and sluggish like a large bag of chips consumed in one sitting does to you? The more you understand how your body reacts to different foods, the better you will be able to nourish it with the best.

For someone with an intolerance or allergy, it is very convenient to hide behind them, but you have to change your behavior as well. Indolence doesn't have to limit you or make you follow a strict diet. In fact, it should open you up to trying foods you never tried before and develop a perception about them. Who knows you end up finding a bunch of foods you never tried before but ended up liking them? Besides, it also prevents feeling food-deprived and leaves with a more inclusive diet.

Take Away

In this chapter, we looked at the many different eating orders, learned about what caused them, pondered over the various symptoms patients depict and later dealt with the most pressing question about intuitive eating — how can someone with dietary restrictions can eat intuitively.

Chapter 6: Becoming an Intuitive Eater

Eating intuitively is becoming a prominent and preferred way of eating today. Much of its hype is due to the fact that diets are failing people and they are finally realizing the harm it does to their body and mind. Be it the Atkins, vegan, keto or the paleo diet, their foundation is based on limitations and restrictions. It gets even worse when you jump from one diet to another simultaneously as it doesn't allow the body to get used to the new change when it had only begun to respond to the changes made prior.

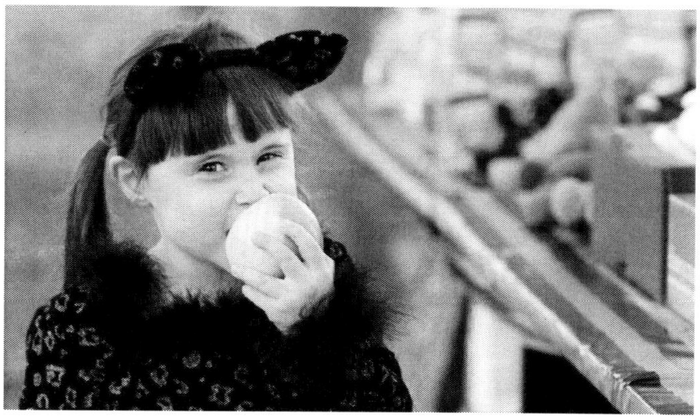

The decision to diet involves more of our mental than our physical body. Who decides what our body needs and what it doesn't? The mind. Add to that societal pressure that keeps on projecting thinness as a beacon of beauty. But even then, it is up to us to decide what is best for us. Our thinking plays a key role.

When people decide to diet, they have a completely different mindset that promotes that thinking. However, since we are more interested in the mindset of an intuitive eater, let's compare both the mentalities and choose which one seems more sane, sustainable and suitable for you.

The Thought Process of an Intuitive Eater and Dieter

A Dieter's Mentality	Issue	An Intuitive Eater's Mentality
Do I Deserve it?	**Food Choices and Eating**	Do I want it? Am I hungry?
I am guilty when I eat fun foods.		Will it satisfy my craving for it?
I describe food as bad and good.		Do I like its taste?
Food is my enemy		I deserve to eat without feeling guilty.
My goal is to burn the calories.	**Benefits of Exercise**	My focus is on how exercise makes me feel.
I feel disappointed when I miss a day at the gym.		My focus isn't on how many days I work out but how energizing and stress-relieving it feels.
Do others think I look good or not?	**Viewing Progress**	I give inner body cues priority.
I have a strong willpower.		I have complete trust in myself and the food that I eat.
How many pounds have I lost?		My primary concern isn't losing weight but eating healthy.

You must have noticed the vast differences between the two mentalities. Firstly, where a dieter is more concerned about losing weight, an intuitive eater just wants to consume food that is healthy and nutritious. Secondly, there is no restriction of food and everything is allowed in an intuitive diet as long as it has good nutritional value and is satisfying. A dieter is rarely concerned about the satisfaction of the consumed food, meaning he or she is eating senselessly and thus depriving the body of not only a variety of nutrition but also taste and satisfaction. Thirdly, a dieter is always thinking about whether he or she should eat something, whereas an intuitive eater lets their body to decide if they want it or not.

If, as suggested by the above table, there is a difference between these two mentalities, then is there a possibility to jump from one to the other? Can a dieter become an intuitive eater if he begins to think like one?

Yes, but it is slightly difficult to change one's mentality completely when they are in adulthood. What were once just random conducts of action have turned into strong habits. Therefore, the only way to challenge them is with hard evidence.

Thus, it is best to start young and teach kids to be intuitive eaters during the developmental stages when they are forming opinions about things, learning, and forming habits.

Raising Intuitive Eaters

As discussed earlier, kids are intuitive eaters by birth. From the moment they are born, they have cried for food and had been fed. Then when they hit toddlerhood and began to differentiate between different foods, their taste, appearance, and smell, they demanded things of their choosing, which was, in fact, their body demanding them. With a few words to describe their needs, they were smart enough to tell their parents what they wanted. And when they felt full, they stopped. As fascinating as it was to watch them munch on their food, it is also important to note their likes and dislikes changed with time, even within hours. For example, has your child ever embarrassed you at a friend's or relative's house by eating something so delightfully that you told your friends and relatives that they hate it? You may have said something like, "Oh, my Timmy hates gummy bears. I tried so hard to get him to eat some but even the colors don't attract him." Moments later, Timmy is trying to fill his little mouth with as many gummy bears as he can fit making you come out as a liar.

However, you weren't a liar and you were right, he didn't like it, until today and that is because "he" felt like having them. Kids love to explore, and their exploration isn't limited to putting their fingers into places they shouldn't be. They are fascinated by their food as well. One day they cry the whole day for some boiled peas and wouldn't even touch one the next day. As parents we think, what the hell, and deliberately try to push them into eating them. What we are doing is taking away their intuitiveness. The ability to decide what their body needs with something that "we" want them to have. It is understandable that as their parents, you want the best for them, but what if we tell you that they are a better judge of it than you are?

Even we as kids were once intuitive eaters. We troubled our parents during feeding times because we weren't hungry, and they were determined to make us eat every last food on the plate. Somewhere in between that, we all grew up. Instead of listening to our bodies, we listened to those who seemed like experts at food and nutrition and changed the way we used to think and feel about our food. And that is when the problem actually began.

Food rules don't always begin at home. They can also form in places other than home such as our schools. Remember the time when the teacher wouldn't allow us to leave the table until we had finished our lunch? And there was a specific time allotted for the break which meant that if you felt extremely hunger before the lunch break, you were allowed to eat food and if you didn't feel hungry during the lunch break, you were still asked to finish your lunch? Sounds unfair, no? Add to that the rewards we were promised. "Honey, if you finish your food, daddy and I will take you out for ice cream. You like ice cream, right?" Bribery worked its magic and despite being full, we were forced to overeat. These are examples of how we have been interfering between our kids and their bodies. We have changed their eating behavior to meet a standard only to realize later, that it was a mistake. So, if it happened with you but you don't want your child to go through the same, below are some great ideas to raise your kid as an intuitive eater and promote behavior that allows them to listen to and put their body needs first.

How to Raise Your Kids to Become Intuitive Eaters?

Be a Good Teacher

Who, according to you is a good teacher? Someone who knows what he or she is doing or someone who is just reading from a book? Someone who believes and lives by the values they teach their kids every day or someone who is just concerned with the end result at the end of the course?

In order to teach your kids how to become an intuitive eater, you must become one first. You have to heal your relationship with food first so that you can know how they will feel and respond to the new changes. Besides, we all know that kids are great imitators. They do as they see others doing. And who are better role models than parents themselves?

Thus, if you want them to eat intuitively, you need to teach them by example. Your kid looks up to you in all aspects of life. So, if they see you restricting yourself from certain foods, they will think of them as distasteful too. Likewise, if you don't feel good about yourself, the way you look, and your food choices, then chances are they too will pick up on the negativity and think of themselves the same way.

When you are around your child, avoid labeling different foods as good or bad. If they want sweets, don't tell them that it will lead to a toothache. If they want a bag of chips, don't scare them by telling them that will cause their stomach to ache. You must remove all feelings of guilt and shame towards foods. Intuitive eating teaches us that there is no such thing as good or bad food, and we must tell them the same as well.

Aim for Balance but Allow Them Options

Allow them to have food with different textures, colors, and shapes. It is all about what sparks the most fascination for a kid. Since they love to explore new things, a variety of things to choose from will make mealtimes more enjoyable for them. Include a combination of fruits and vegetables or nuts and dairy. And don't get upset when they eat some of the things on their plate and leave others. What better insight would you have than knowing of their preference? If you are trying to make them an intuitive eater, you just need to add more of the things they ate the next time around, even if they weren't the most nutritious of foods. Intuitive eating doesn't restrict any foods and the different combinations will only make it easier for you to understand what your child likes and doesn't like.

Don't Stop Offering

Gaining a preference over their favorite foods is going to be a long process. Think of the foods as reality show contestants. They all have their own skills and talents, but it is only the judge that chooses the best out of them and says bye to the remaining one. Try offering your kids something new every day so that they can pick. The key is to never stop offering something new or intentionally placing on their plates, the foods that were rejected the last time. Although it is a nice tactic, it doesn't guarantee results. What if your kid eats it now because he or she is super hungry but doesn't even look at it the next time because they have other things on their plate too.

Another important thing for parents to know is to encourage the use of words like crunchy, sour, sweet, and soupy to describe food. The next time you ask them, and they tell you that they want crunchy, give them foods that fit that description. This will encourage them to eat when foods are grouped into different categories. To make things more interesting, try presenting it in playful ways such as assorted by color or arranged in different shapes or placed on the plate according to their sizes. Not only will it make their mealtime more interesting, but it will also be something that they can learn from.

Mind Your Language Around Food

How you speak about different foods is important as kids pick up things very fast. Labeling things as good or bad will only lead the kids into thinking about them in a judgmental way. Instead, try using words like fun foods or growing foods instead of junk food or healthy foods. Since your goal is to make them an intuitive eater, labeling something as bad will add a negative connotation to it.

Let Them Be the Judge

As parents, we all want to offer our kids the best that is out there. However, sometimes we feel like despite their favorite things being placed right in front of them, they seem disinterested. You keep trying to push them into eating and they do take a few bites, but it seems more forceful than enjoyable. Let your kids choose when they want to eat and what they want to eat. Trying to force the idea that they are somehow bound by a time constraint is wrong. Have you ever eaten a big meal for lunch and didn't feel like eating dinner? The reason you didn't eat at dinner time is because your intuition told you that you weren't hungry. The same thing happens with kids. They are born with the same intuition, so let them use it wisely.

Conversely, if a kid keeps on asking for something every few hours, then don't shush them and tell them they can't have it now because there is only an hour left for dinner. Kids are experts in their own bodies. Maybe the previous meal they ate was digested faster. Perhaps they had a busy and active day and thus their body needs some more energy to keep going. The point here is, don't question their motives for eating. If they say they are hungry, they probably are. The same applies to when they tell you that they have eaten enough. Don't try to force-feed them what's left on their plate or in their bowl.

Lastly, if they have a bad feeling towards certain vegetables, don't force them to eat them. This will set a negative connotation towards those vegetables and your child will always throw a tantrum when they are presented again. Of course, your intentions are to feed them with good nutrition but let that be for some other day or time.

The Holiday Survival Guide When Eating Intuitively

Holidays are that time of the year when we are bombarded with texts from friends and family, planning our holiday dinners, and checking our availability. However, you just starting intuitively. How are you going to handle the delicious starters, the devour-able entrees, and the sweetest of desserts? You already had a little too much around Halloween and swore that you wouldn't get into that eating frenzy ever again. What are you going to do to control your eating when literally everyone is insisting that you take some more?

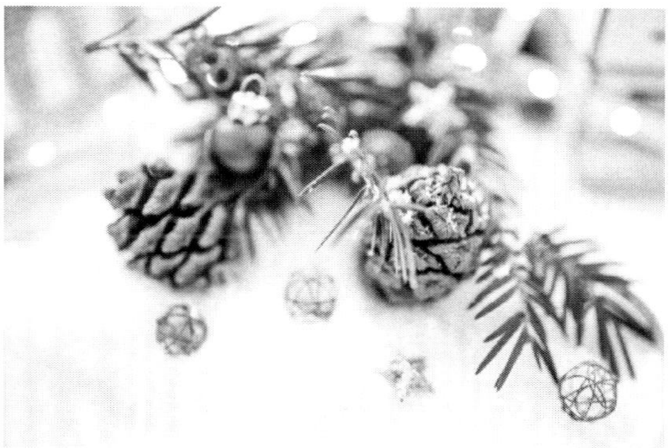

Well, for starters, intuitive eating has never stopped you from eating the things you love. Of course, there are a few limitations like stopping when you are full but that doesn't mean you ditch the desserts variety completely. There are multiple ways to manage your cravings around food, even during the Holidays.

Most of us fall for the old dieting patterns thinking we will be eating too much around the holidays and gaining weight. True, there is this possibility and also that no matter how hard you try, you will still be tempted by everything that is presented in front of you. So are you going to worry about your weight or miss out on the delicacies until next year?

To help a diva like you in distress, we are presenting you with a number of ways you can keep eating intuitively without having to worry about gaining a few extra pounds here and there. Keep in mind that this time of the year is supposedly the most joyous one and your body deserves a treat too.

Visualize

Visualize how you are going to spend your time during the holidays. Think about what you will be wearing, who you will be talking to, how you will respond to food, how much you will eat, and how you will feel after eating it. The more detailed your visualization, the more prepared you will be to live that moment. Think of it as a rehearsal before an actual event. It only makes you more confident and in control.

What visualization will do here is to get your mind off of food and the worry associated with it. When you have a little plan of action about how you are going to approach food, how much you are going to eat, and how it will feel when you have it, it will make it less focusable. You will then be more concerned about meeting your family and friends and enjoy your time with them. You won't worry about whether you need to go for a run the very next day or not. Instead, you can act a little relaxed because you have it all under control.

We are most worried when we are faced with an uncertain situation – something we didn't plan for. However, thanks to visualization, the stress around food and whether you will be able to control will be minimized and prevent any emotional eating.

Create a Few Mantras

Next, you need to create a few mantras of your own to get you by the holiday season. Whether you like it or not, there will be someone discussing a new diet they found extremely helpful to shed weight or a new drink or supplement that makes you cut down on food, so you won't feel hungry all day. It is unavoidable and likely to make you impatient for two reasons. First, you are eating intuitively which means there is no restriction or limitation to what you can eat and second, you will be worried that your intuitive approach towards eating will be mocked and laughed at because it is not a diet, just normal eating. But remember, how you respond is up to you. You can either feel bad about your eating habits or completely dismiss their eating approach. So, every time you are faced with some backlash or forced into a conversation about food, chant to yourself something like,

"I don't need to listen to this" or "It doesn't concern me, I should keep doing what I am doing." Doing so will serve as a reminder that you aren't wrong and don't have to listen to some gibberish all night just because you reject the diet mentality.

Secondly, you might also come across people who wouldn't stop gloating about how much miles they jog every day and that you should definitely try it sometime too. There is no forcing in intuitive eating. You aren't in a herd. You won't do what everyone else is doing. You will jog the day you feel like it, and more importantly, when your body feels like it. Again chant your mantras in your head and you will reassure yourself that you are doing well for yourself and your body.

Focus Your Energy and Time Elsewhere

Again, if you keep all your focus on what you are going to eat and how you are going to control and stop when you're full, then you will miss out on all that is happening. If the thoughts of food still haunt you, try distracting yourself by conversing with people. The more involved you are in the conversation, the less likely you are going to think about food. Thus, try engaging with people as it will help you drown out the voice in your brain worried about whether it will be chaos when the food is served or not.

Your goal should be to respond to food and not just react. You need to eat mindfully and not just try everything out of fear. And when the food is finally served, use the opposite strategy and avoid any conversations as it will only take your mind off of how much you have actually eaten, and you will miss your internal cues for when you are full.

Note That Feeling Little Too Full Is Acceptable

If, however, for some reason you do end up overeating, there is no need to start panicking. You haven't broken any rules. You just have eaten a little beyond your fullness. Intuitive eating is also about experiencing foods and if something feels so good that you have to request for seconds, don't regret it later. If it was worth it, then there is no point stressing about it. Don't start planning your next workout routine or promising yourself that you would skip all the following events until you have burned the extra calories. More importantly, don't give up on eating intuitively thinking you aren't worth it. It is okay to go over your eating intake. It's not like you will gain weight in a single sitting. Stressing will only mess up your mood and mental health.

Allow Yourself to Eat

Lastly, you have permission to eat. You need to verbally remind yourself of that, especially when you are trying to hold back onto something. Remember, you aren't following a diet anymore and have the liberty to eat whatever you feel like eating, even if that means stuffing yourself with stuffed chicken with oozing cheese. You have to allow yourself to enjoy food without judgment, otherwise, there is no point in eating it. Tell your body that it is allowed to eat whatever it craves, any time it wants, and until it feels full. Doing so will take the regret out of food and make your holidays less stressful and more enjoyable for you.

Take Away

In this chapter, we looked at the many different aspects of intuitive eating starting from the differences between the two mentalities — a dieter's and an intuitive eater. After stressing on the need for intuitive eating, we later delved into how parents can raise kids that are intuitive eaters and avoid the mistakes they usually make.

Lastly, as a bonus, we looked at how one can carry themselves during the holiday season which tends to be the most exhausting for anyone who has just started to eat intuitively. The practices include everything from distracting yourself from food to accepting that it is okay to eat without guilt and shame.

Chapter 7: Intuitive Eating and Weight Loss

Unlike any diet, the core essence of intuitive eating isn't weight loss. It is more about addressing the different ways we eat. So, if someone has had a positive reduction in their weight with intuitive eating, good for them. But that doesn't mean everyone will feel the same or be greeted with the same outcome.

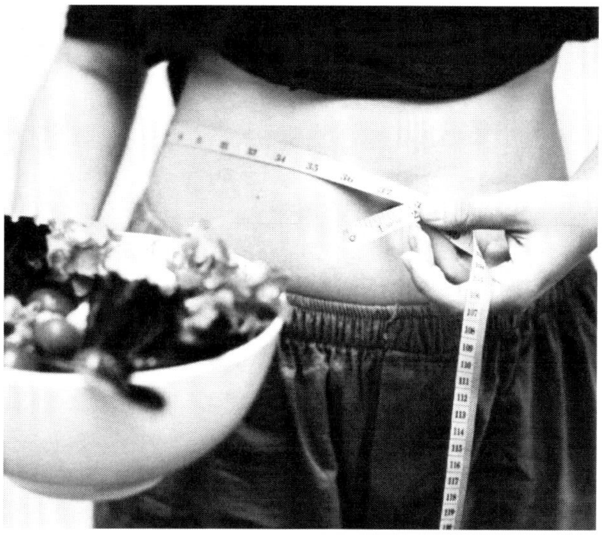

Although the possibility of intuitive eating leading to weight loss is still debated and there are different schools of thought. Since it is a fairly new way of eating, there is still room for more research and experiments to confirm this hypothesis. In this chapter, we are going to be discussing some of the most prominent and promising research studies and experiments that prove that intuitive eating does have promising results when it comes to one's weight maintenance, body image satisfaction, higher self-esteem, and better emotional functioning.

How Listening to Your Body Can Help You Lose Weight?

Traditional dieting programs have proven ineffective in promising sustainable results in the long run. It is quite common that lost weight is gained in less time once the dieting stops and the restrictions are uplifted. And that isn't even the worst part about them. They also happen to leave behind multiple psychological traumas such as anxiety regarding food, binge and emotional eating, and feelings of guilt and shame later. Such eating patterns are no good to anyone, especially someone who is trying to reestablish their relationship with food.

According to a study published in the *Journal of the Academy of Nutrition and Dietetics* titled *A Review of Interventions that Promote Eating* by Internal Cues, researchers, Magnuson and Schafer, reviewed all the former studies around intuitive eating. All quasi-experimental controlled trials, randomized controlled trials, and cohort studies were reviewed. The goal of the research evaluation was to determine whether internal hunger and fullness cues, pleasure, satiety played any key role in weight management, weight loss or developing a healthier relationship with food or not.

The authors further reviewed all articles containing the terms intuitive eating, non-diet, mindful eating, attuned eating, and even health at every size intervention approach to eating.

After a thorough study of each and later selecting only the most relevant studies, the authors found 24 studies and articles that were later included in their final review. As per their findings, it was collectively concluded that patients who were previously obese or overweight and then looked at intuitive eating as a savior did report significant decreases in their weight.

According to a 2013 report published in the *Journal Appetite* by National Eating Disorder Association, approximately half a million young adults suffer from disordered eating and disrupted sleeping patterns which affected their skin, body functions, and energy levels. The most prominently observed disorders included compulsive eating, emotional eating, restrictive eating, obsession with certain foods, etc. Surprisingly, when a sample of 2,287 teenagers was studied, the researchers tried to study their eating habits. It was revealed that those who let their hunger cues determine their need for food intake were less likely to fall into the despair of eating disorders. They also reported better sleeping patterns and elevated energy levels compared to those who listened more to external cues than their own.

A research paper published in the *American Journal of Health Education* studied the meaning of food, the role of intuitive eating, and the relationship with the two versus diet composition. Intuitive eating proved to be a viable and sustainable approach to maintaining a healthy weight. The research survey included 343 university students who were asked their opinion regarding the intuitive eating scale and other diet-related scales. These were the conclusions drawn after an evaluation of their answers.

- Students that scored higher on the hunger and fullness (intuitive scale) reported lower BMI.
- Students who scored higher on the hunger and fullness scale also reported being less health-conscious when it comes to their relationship with food.
- Students who scored higher on the hunger and fullness scale also seemed to value the pleasure that comes from eating and food and reported higher levels of satisfaction.

To conclude, those individuals who gave their inner cues more value reported a healthier relationship with food and were less concerned about their weight management as compared to those who had been dieting. They also reported less anxiety around food and cared less about calories and more about how the food made them feel.

In another study published in the *Journal of American Dietetic Association*, researchers tried to figure out if intuitive eating helped one deal with size-related issues and led to the acceptance of the way they looked or not. The objective of the research was to determine how effective health at every size approach was and whether it helped people in improving their health or not.

Health at every size serves as an encouragement to eat intuitively and develop homeostasis regulation. A group of 78 females who were in the obese category were called upon to participate in a study. All of them were chronic dieters in their 30s and 40s. They were all asked to attend a six-month program including weekly intervention called the Diet Program vs. Health at Every Size Program. The clinical trial was followed by a six-month aftercare support group.

Throughout the study, the following measures were evaluated:

- Anthropometry
- Metabolic fitness
- Eating behavior
- Energy expenditure
- Attrition
- Psychology
- Participation and attendance in the study

It was noted that attrition was the highest in the diet group being 41%, whereas there was only 8% in the health at every size group. After the intervention, the diet group did show some swift improvements in multiple variables; however, it was only short-lived. In fact, they regained the weight they had lost and the improvements they had shown weren't sustained in the coming years.

On the contrary, the health at every size group not only maintained their weight in the next two years, but they also showed sustainability in the overall improved variables. So to conclude, it can be said more promising results were observed in those who had health at every size approach towards eating. The changes they made over time with intuitive eating were far more sustainable in the long run.

Another groundbreaking study consisting of different groups of teenagers proposed that intuitive eating can lower the risk of developing eating disorders like binge eating, midnight snacking, and emotional eating and also alleviate their symptoms. Compared with traditional means of dieting, which only makes one more worried about their calorie intake, this serves as a refreshing reminder that those battling eating disorders can switch to intuitive eating to prevent their onset and progression. Disordered eating has been reported to increase one's risk of developing multiple health conditions including blood pressure, stroke, obesity, and digestive problems. It also has a psychological impact and linked to increased anxiety and depression in many.

Although it is too early to say, intuitive eating does have many perks that no other eating approach offers. But of course, more research needs to go into finding how it actually works and how it can be adopted as the only approach to eating healthy.

Chapter 8: Intuitive Eating FAQs

As someone trying out intuitive eating for the first time, there must be many boggling questions on your mind regarding this non-diet mentality and whether this is the right approach for you or not, especially if you have been dieting religiously and just looking for an alternative approach this time around. Luckily, in this chapter, we are going to be answering some of the most pressing and obvious FAQs regarding intuitive eating for those in search of them.

So without further ado, let's get answering!

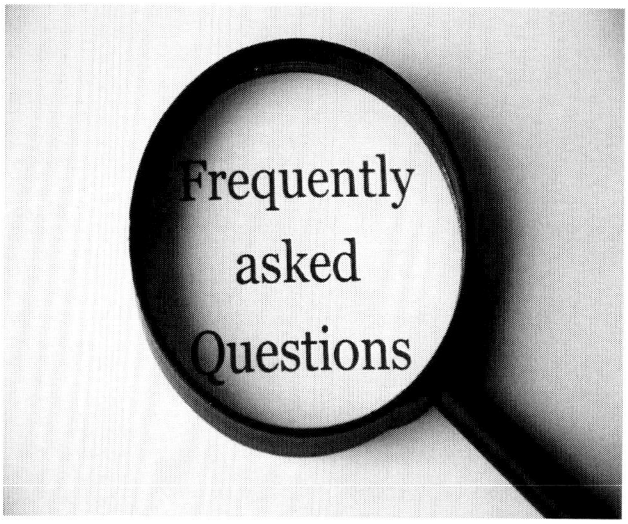

Is IE a Diet?

Sadly, no!

Instead, intuitive eating is a response to the diet mentality that strongly opposes the diet culture. There are no stringent rules and regulations that you must follow but there are 10 principles that teach you how to practice intuitive eating. The term was coined by two California-based dieticians Evelyn Tribole and Emily Resch, who after dealing with many diet-focused clients decided to publish their findings to help people get over the diet culture and focus more on building a sustainable relationship with food.

Where all diets tell you to abstain from a certain food group, there is no such limitation in eating intuitively. You also don't have to restrain yourself from any cravings you might have as intuitive eating allows its followers to consume whatever they like, in whatever quantity they like and whenever they like. This recognition of zero food rules is what makes it so unique from any other diet in the world and thus more doable. The majority of the work required to eat intuitively is to give up the former rules you abided by when you were dieting, which is easier said than done but possible.

Am I doing it right?

If you are treating intuitive eating as a diet, then there is a chance that you are doing it wrong. Here are some of the signs that you need to change your approach and start eating right.

- If you still feel like you have to hold yourself back from certain foods, then you are doing it wrong. Intuitive dieting is against restrictive eating behaviors.
- If you are still worried about the calories in everything and counting them mentally before every meal, then you are not eating intuitively. You need to stop focusing on the calories in everything and enjoy it. Also when you are too focused on counting the calories, there is a possibility that you won't be able to spot your hunger cues and overeat.
- If you are calculating the results by weighing yourself daily, then you aren't eating right. Intuitive eating is more about sustainable weight than weight loss. True, it does help some lose weight, but it isn't the actual goal. So, if you started eating intuitively thinking it will help you shed a few pounds and get you in shape, then you began with the wrong idea and may be disappointed with the results.

Does it Work?

It comes down to your definition of the word "work." What was the goal you began with when you first started eating intuitively? Was it to build a healthy relationship with your food or was it to lose weight? One of the biggest dilemmas with intuitive eating is that people measure their success by the weight they lost rather than an improvement in their eating habits. They think that as long as some diet is allowing them to lose weight, it means it is working and vice versa.

Intuitive eating is more concerned about listening to your body's needs and leading a happy and mentally strong life free from guilt, shame or judgment of any kind. If this fits your criteria for what you mean by "working," then yes it works remarkably well.

What if I also want to lose weight? Is it ideal for me then?

If weight loss is your ultimate goal, then it may or may not help you.

As stated above, intuitive eating is more of a philosophy than a diet that encourages us to pay attention to our body's needs. It preaches to us to look for inner cues and schedule our meals. It promotes satisfaction that can only come from enjoying our meals to the fullest. It tells us to stop eating when we are full and never indulge in unnecessary overeating. It reminds us that it is okay to crave certain foods and that we mustn't deprive our bodies of them.

So, to say whether it will affect you or not and help you lose your desired weight is a very difficult and personalized question. Even the diets we follow demonstrate different results on different body types. Some people only lose water weight, while others are down by 10 pounds.

Since the goal of intuitive dieting is to break the chain of endless diets and take people out of their miseries of rollercoaster diets, it is very hard to tell if it will help them lose weight or not. There may also be times where you feel like you are gaining weight rather than losing it with intuitive eating. So, it is a matter of personal choice, to be honest. Ask yourself this, would you rather feel miserable and count every last calorie or would you like to stop worrying about that once and for all and stop skipping between different diets?

Your answer will determine if it is for you or not.

I fear that I will only eat junk if I start eating intuitively. How will I be able to stop?

Again, this is a very genuine concern that most people switching from a restrictive diet to intuitive eating is worried about it. True, this will be difficult but only because you are coming from a place where everything, but a few things were restricted. So, your first instinct would be to eat all the things that were once forbidden to your heart's content. There is also a chance that you won't stop eating even when you are full because you are so overwhelmed with how it is making you feel. This happens because your body has waited long enough to taste it and thus sends interrupted cues.

Secondly, after some time you will realize that you no longer feel the craving. Ask yourself would you like to have a donut on the seventh day as well as after the meal? If yes, would it still give you the same satisfaction it did on the first day you had it after so many weeks or months? Probably not! It is because you didn't hold yourself back from it and allowed your body to enjoy it as much as possible. However, after some time the body begins to see it as monotonous and craves something else.

To answer your question if you will ever stop craving junk and eat healthily, then yes. You will although it will take some time to adjust to the new eating approach, so stay patient and don't lose hope.

Do I have to be driven?

Unlike any diet, there are no days, set timings or a list of things you can and can't eat. When you are bound by time and a number of days, you are more likely to stick around and feel motivated. It is the same as having a deadline to submit a report. When you take out that deadline you will possibly delay working on the report until the very last minute. Since there is an absence of a deadline or ultimate goal with intuitive eating, many may suffer from a lack of motivation, to begin with. Since it is eating like you normally would and everything you can, it can take some time to grow on you and make you want to continue with it. Until then, take your time and be patient. Even if you suffer from a lack of motivation, try not to give up and continue eating intuitively.

How will I know when I am hungry and when I am full? Is there some particular way to judge my fullness?

There is no secret formula to listening to your inner cues. You just need to practice and practice. We have already talked about the hunger and fullness scale. Try to place your level of hunger on it and see if you really are hungry or can still wait a few hours before eating something. The same applies to identify your fullness. Think of one on the scale as ravenous, four as neutral and 10 as full. The numbers may represent your hunger and fullness differently, but since you are just starting out, it is best to start with this. You can always adjust your numbers on the scale later based on your own preference. Also, each number is going to affect you differently. For instance, at level three, you may feel a growling tummy, but your friend might feel lightheaded. So everyone's scale is different. Moreover, it is best to avoid taking your hunger to a one as it may make you extremely hungry and you might end up overeating. Therefore, you must practice mindfulness at all times because the fullness cues are easy to miss. And Since the goal is to stop eating when you're full, you don't want to overeat and later regret it.

Lastly, let patience be your guide. It will take some time before you are able to exactly guess your hunger or fullness level. This is extremely hard for those who have been on restrictive diets as their hunger and fullness scale is messed up. But there is no need to be too harsh on yourself as it will only lead to losing your motivation and giving up on intuitive eating altogether.

How long before I become an intuitive eater?

This is a very subjective question as everyone's progress will be different. We all have our own timelines. You may have a hard time getting over something, while your friend may get over it in a few days or weeks. It all comes down to how well or poorly you react to change and how long you've been dieting for. The more damaged your relationship with food is, the longer it will take you to adapt to this approach. But even then, there is always a possibility of going back to your old practices, which means you will have to start from scratch altogether.

So, there can't be a definitive answer to this. However, if you stay true to yourself, allow your body to cue your hunger and fullness and abide by the 10 principles of intuitive eating, you will be astonished to see how quickly you are progressing towards a healthier lifestyle. Just keep in mind that since it isn't a diet, there isn't any expiration date or time.

If I am only eating junk what about my nutrition?

Believe it or not, there is a great likelihood that you will begin to eat more of what's nutritious and less of what is junk food. How will that happen? Picture this, you had a bowl full of mac and cheese only to realize that it made your tummy bloated and gassy. It isn't a nice feeling and if anything, the satisfaction you experienced while having it is minimized. Contrarily, if you had a bowl full of fruits or veggies, you are likely to feel lighter and more energized. Isn't that a better feeling than being bloated and gassy?

When you analyze the difference, you will want to eat healthier on your own so that you can avoid feeling uncomfortable later, even when the nutritious foods don't taste that good.

I have decided to eat intuitively but where do I begin?

First of all, congratulations to you for making the right decision to value your intuition to guide you from this point onwards. In order to begin, you must become familiar with the 10 principles of intuitive eating which form the basis of it. Secondly, you can seek help from a community of intuitive eaters and share your fears, struggles, and goals to feel like a part of a community. It is a fact that when people work in unison, they are likelier to achieve their goals. Besides, joining a community online or a support group can help you feel less stressed as you will always have someone to answer your questions and realize that you aren't the only one dealing with a particular issue.

There are also many books on intuitive eating which not only promotes the practice but also provides valuable insight on how to begin with the approach. Getting your hands on one of them can be extremely beneficial.

Take Away

In this chapter, we looked at the most commonly asked questions about intuitive eating. The answers are extremely helpful for someone still having a hard time deciding whether they should eat intuitively or take up another diet.

Well, look no further as this chapter answers all your queries in a detailed manner and help you get started with eating intuitively.

Chapter 9: The Benefits of IE

With over a hundred research studies swearing by its effectiveness, in this chapter, we are going to be talking about the benefits of intuitive eating — both the obvious and less obvious ones.

One Step Towards a Healthier You!

The biggest advantages of following the intuitive eating approach as opposed to any restrictive diet include:

- Decreased cholesterol
- Improved eating behaviors
- Decreased blood pressure
- Decreased body dissatisfaction
- Increased physical activity
- Increased self-esteem

These were some scientific researched benefits. Now coming to the less obvious benefits that most people fail to notice when introducing themselves to intuitive eating include:

You Are Able to Honor and Detect Hunger Cues

The best thing about intuitive eating is that it teaches us the art to detect our hunger cues so that we only eat when hunger strikes. This is a great way to honor the body. You are no longer restrained by time or eating mindlessly. You only eat when your body tells you to, even if it is right after you had a meal or late at night. Therefore, you must trust those cues and honor your body with what it craves.

You Are Able to Differentiate Between Foods

Since you aren't permitted to let your external cues decide what you should eat and when, you are no longer a captive to your own body and can feed it with whatever feels good. Since it isn't unlike any other diet, you have a free hand at exploring different food groups and eat things of your liking. With intuitive eating, there aren't any forbidden foods that also cut down your need to binge eat, you did in the past. When all your cravings are met in a timely manner, you no longer feel deprived or eat more than you should which helps with maintaining your weight.

As you explore further, you realize that there are no good or bad foods and that each food has some purpose to serve. This also means that you can enjoy whatever foods you previously didn't know about or restricted yourself from.

You Become Less Guilty About Your Food Choices

There are less guilty feelings surrounding your food. You are able to put the food police to a quiet and eat without being worried about the consequences or how much exercise you will have to do just so that you can burn the calories you've just eaten. There is little to no judgment on your part as well. Doing all this allows you to actually taste your food and feel the effects it has on you.

Food Feels Better to You

When the feelings of guilt, shame or judgment are put to rest, you are finally able to enjoy your food as you should. You begin to eat more mindfully and give all your senses a treat every time you have a meal.

You Become More Aware

As soon as you begin to enjoy your food, you also start noticing the effects of different foods and how they make you feel. Some foods may leave you feeling bloated, while others just uplift and energize your mood. Once you are able to differentiate between food choices like that, you are more likely to eat foods that make you feel happier and elated rather than those that cause bloating and fatigue. This enables you to have a better and healthier relationship with food as you also become aware of your satiety cues.

You Don't Crave Things Like You Used To

This is probably the biggest advantage of intuitive eating. You are able to control and manage your cravings. Since the process of reestablishing trust with your body has begun, you are better able to honor your hunger and fullness by giving your body the things it really wants to eat. This means that you eat what your body requires which makes the onset of cravings less frequent. How? You are no longer restricting yourself from anything.

You Become More Confident About Food Choices

Your self-confidence also takes a boost. When you have established a healthy relationship with your body, minimized the guilt and shame and presented yourself with the opportunity to eat whatever you feel like, you become more confident about yourself. You realize that food is no longer the only thing that defines you and even if it is, then you have it covered. Life is no longer apologetic, and you learn to live it to the fullest. You no longer feel like someone else should be the judge of how you look or should look.

You Become Flexible

For any dieter, it can be both annoying and worrying when they are pushed to show restraint when they are with their friends or peers and forced to just take a break from their diet for just one night. Call it a hardcore dieter's biggest nightmare. Luckily, if you are practicing intuitive eating, you don't have to go through such dilemmas, and you are more open to accepting unplanned dinners and hangouts without feeling any guilt about them later.

You Begin to Enjoy Exercise

Since you are following all the principles of intuitive eating, you are also honoring your body with the right amount of physical exercise to keep it healthy and flexible. When you aren't worried about the numbers on a scale and just exercising because you want to, it stops feeling like a chore and becomes more enjoyable. The moment you realize that you are doing it to please your own body and not anyone else, the workout becomes enjoyable and less stressful. This happens because you begin to view exercise as a means of self-care and not a fat-burning regime. Therefore, if it ever happens that you aren't able to go to the gym or feel like taking a rest day, you won't feel any guilt or shame.

You Are Able to Enjoy Trigger Foods

Wait, did we just say trigger foods? All dieters must be losing their minds and turning pages because now they are craving one. This isn't the case with intuitive eaters as they are not only able to keep them in the house, they can also enjoy them whenever they like. However, since they have excelled at keeping their cravings at bay, there is no hurry to binge eat it all in a single sitting. Sometimes they even forget they have them in the first place which is a prime example of managing cravings.

You Are Able to Stop When You Are Full

No longer do you have to finish everything on the plate once you sense that you have reached the state of fullness. There is no longer any shame in leaving leftovers on the plate as you don't have any obligation to finish it all.

You Are Less Judgmental and More Curious

You begin to approach different foods with more curiosity and less judgment. You don't always have a mental battle with yourself about whether you should have it or not. Instead, you become more thoughtful and reflective. You take full responsibility for your actions and realize that you no longer have to beat yourself up about it or regret it later.

You Become More Receptive

You start trying foods you never tried before. This also includes all those foods you had restricted yourself from eating formerly. You are also more open and receptive to various cuisines. Think of it as trying out a random dish on a restaurant menu instead of scrolling through the menu online and counting the calories in each dish or wearing revealing and fitted clothes because you don't care what everyone is going to think. If you've reached this point in your life, then this is when you have fully adopted intuitive eating.

You Are Less Critical of Yourself

You learn of self-compassion and understand how important it is to feel comfortable in your own skin. You no longer are worried about losing weight or looking good in a dress; your prime concerns become enjoying your time and feeling the freedom that comes with intuitive eating. You also start caring for yourself and treat yourself with things you previously were too afraid to even try. Alternatively, you also stop beating yourself up about the way you look or how others see you and just feel like "you."

You Turn to Coping Mechanisms Other Than Food

What once was the easiest option is no longer an option anymore. While eating intuitively, you realize how damaging it was to eat mindlessly, driven by emotions and cravings. They no longer remain a viable coping mechanism as you know that giving in to the temptation of food will only make you regret it later and cause health concerns. Therefore, when a craving does arise or you are down with emotions, you look for other ways to overcome them instead of relying solely on food.

You Feel More Elated

There is a significant improvement in your mood. Since you have successfully eliminated all the guilt and shame associated with food, you no longer are fearful about your cravings or eating things that were once restricted. You become more concerned about how you feel physically and mentally and in general feel happier and satisfied with your choices.

You Feel Satisfied

In general, your life stops revolving around food, which means you have more space in your head to think about the other things happening around you. When you find yourself becoming an active part of conversations, you get good at relationships with others. This only adds to your satisfaction with your life as you are able to focus your mind and energy elsewhere. There is little stress or worry about what others think of you or the way you look which boosts your self-confidence and promotes happiness.

You Become Mindful

Mindfulness and intuitive eating go hand in hand. As soon as you begin to eat intuitively, you also become a mindful eater. There are hundreds of benefits of each and when you are practicing both at a time, you can imagine how many advantages you are able to get. You become more aware of the present and focus on what you are eating right now instead of worrying about your next meal. This also leads to more self-awareness about your body and you become better at addressing your internal cues.

Take Away

This chapter looked at the various ways of how eating mindfully can help us from lowering our cholesterol and blood pressure levels to promoting eating mindfully. It helps us improve our perception on how we look and helps us enjoy exercising. It also reminds us to cope with our emotions and feelings with things other than food to ensure us that trigger foods will no longer trigger us... All of this and much more have been discussed in this chapter to help you learn of the multitude of benefits IE offers.

Chapter 10: Is it For Me?

This is one of the most pressing questions everyone planning to make the big switch ask themselves every day. Although we have covered most of it in the FAQ section, if you still have a few doubts, here is our final answer to this.

Who Benefits the Most from Intuitive Eating?

If you are looking for a one-word answer then here it is — EVERYONE!*

*Of course, there are a few exceptions such as those who are diabetic or suffer from some other severe health issues like Crohn's disease. But then again, no other diet is good for them either as they can't simply eat whatever their gut tells them to. Other than that, some of the groups of people that can benefit the most with intuitive dieting include:

Dieters: Those who have or still choose to the diet can reap great benefits with intuitive eating. Since they mostly have to practice restriction with certain foods, they can get rid of them once and for all with intuitive eating.

Kids: Being naturally intuitive, kids growing up as intuitive eaters can be more in control with their eating behaviors and less likely to develop an eating disorder if they have been taught to eat intuitively from an early age.

Teenagers: Teenagers or college-goers are the biggest age group battling with eating disorders. The disorders arise due to several inappropriate eating habits such as binge eating, snacking up too much on fun foods, and interrupted sleeping patterns. Intuitive eating principles can help them build a better and more promising eating behavior as they grow older and step into the professional world, which, let's face it, is only going to be harder and more draining. Therefore, the possibility of neglecting food or adopting good food habits is rare.

Workaholics: Workaholics have a severed relationship with food. Their eating is usually clocked and consists of basically whatever they can get their hands on. There is no structure to their diets which can lead to multiple health conditions later in life. How can they benefit from eating intuitively? By listening to their inner cues and taking out the time to care for their body and mind by giving it some nutrition and rest.

Obese or Overweight: One of the biggest challenges to losing weight is abstaining from former habits. Since people who are obese have no rules to eating, this is the first thing they need to work on when they are trying to get in shape. How can intuitive eating help in doing so? Well, if you are looking for an answer now, you really have missed all the advice we served you within this book. Go back to the 10 principles and tell us that they aren't enough to motivate you to reassess your eating habits? As soon as you start eating intuitively, you will notice a change in your urge for foods and with time, you will realize that food isn't the only thing on your mind anymore. When that gets settled in, you will move forward with honoring your body and only indulge in foods that are gentle nutrition. And as soon as you start honoring your body, listening to the hunger cues and stopping when full will become easier.

Binge or Emotional Eaters: Lastly, binge or emotional eaters can benefit from intuitive eating as well. Since their primary way of responding to any situation, be it good or bad, is with food, limiting the amount they eat in short intervals of time or eating too much at a time can help them get back to having a healthy relationship with food and also help them get back in shape.

Intuitive eating is for everyone looking to build a healthy relationship with food. There are no exceptions whatsoever and everyone can reap the remarkable advantages it has to offer.

Conclusion

At first, the idea of using your intuition to help you figure out an eating approach best for you may seem scary and downright ridiculous. But you mustn't forget that we all were once intuitive eaters. It is all about going back to your roots and starting afresh, how nature wanted it to be like originally. As kids, we let our intuition and curiosity guide us and as it turns out, we did grow up to be good and healthy, then why fear to listen to it again? We ate when we were hungry, rejected eating more when full, enjoyed eating a few things and rejected the ones we didn't. Simple no?

It wasn't until we were indoctrinated and introduced to the diet culture popularized by a few big brands who one day decided to take control of our eating habits. Add to that the obsession with thinness and how it affected the lives of millions across the globe trying to eat in a restrictive way so that they can look a certain way.

Thankfully, with the advent of intuitive eating, we again have a chance to turn back time and eat like we were supposed to. So are you going to take that chance or not?

We hope that this book offers all the insights you had been craving for related to intuitive eating. It has the potential to make your life fulfilling, happier and more satisfactory. It has everything — a guide to starting out, the 10 principles to lead you, answers to all your mind-boggling questions and myths that needed to be debunked and how you can implement the approach to intuitive eating into your life.

Finally, if you enjoyed this book, then I'd like to ask you if you would you be kind enough to leave a review for this book on Amazon? It would be greatly appreciated!

>> Scan with your camera to leave a quick review:

Thank you and I can't wait to see your thoughts.

YOUR FREE GIFTS

As a way of saying thanks for your purchase and to help you along your journey towards developing healthier eating habits, we've created free bonus resources that will help you get the best possible results:

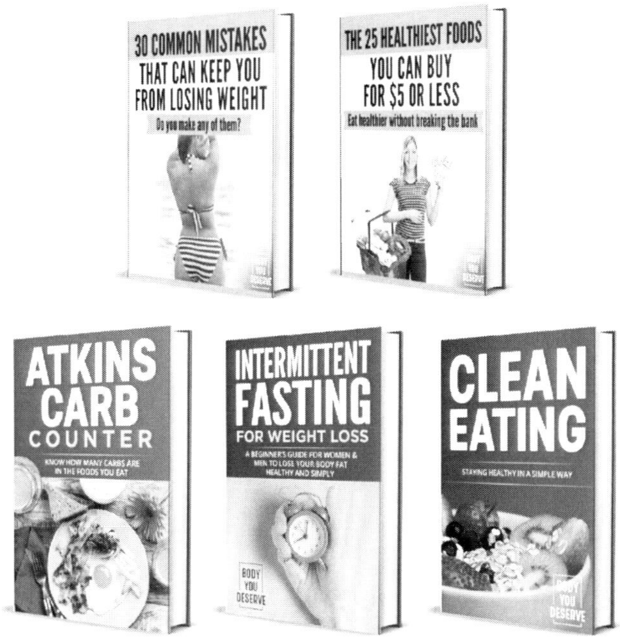

Free bonus #1: 30 Common mistakes that can keep you from losing weight
Do you make any of them?

Free bonus #2: The 25 Healthiest Foods You Can Buy for $5 or Less
Eat healthier without breaking the bank

Free bonus #3: Atkins carb counter
Know how many carbs are in the foods you eat

Free bonus #4: Intermittent Fasting for Weight Loss
A beginners guide for women & men to lose your body fat healthy and simply

Free bonus #5: Clean Eating
Staying healthy in a simple way

To get your bonuses, go to: http://bit.ly/NathalieSeaton

or scan with your camera:

References

10 Principles of Intuitive Eating. (n.d.). Retrieved from https://www.intuitiveeating.org/10-principles-of-intuitive-eating/

Abbate, E. (2019). 4 Reasons Diets Don't Work (And Never Will). Retrieved from https://www.shape.com/weight-loss/tips-plans/why-you-should-stop-restrictive-dieting

Bodak, C. (2017). 6 different types of eaters: Which one are you? Retrieved from https://www.fox19.com/story/34630196/6-different-types-of-eaters-which-one-are-you/

Graue, L. (2019). An exploration of differences between intuitive eating and mindful eating. Retrieved from https://www.fiercelyembodied.com/blog/an-exploration-of-differences-between-intuitive-eating-and-mindful-eating

Grabinsky, C., Matthews, D., Arnold, C., Marvel, P., Jure, J., & Cantwell, E. (2015). THE BROWNIE EXPERIMENT.

Harbstreet, C. (2019). What to Do About the Holidays When You're Working on Intuitive Eating. Retrieved from http://www.streetsmartnutrition.com/intuitive-eating-for-holidays/

Lauren Fowler. (2015). Intuitive Eating 101: How to Get Started. Retrieved from https://www.laurenfowler.co/blog/intuitive-eating-101

Malacoff, J., & Malacoff, J. (n.d.). Why Intuitive Eating Is Actually Really Difficult. Retrieved from https://www.shape.com/healthy-eating/diet-tips/intuitive-eating-problems-tips

Miller, K. (n.d.). The Real Reason You Don't Need A Diet. Retrieved from https://www.refinery29.com/en-us/diet-problems

Morrot, G., Brochet, F., & Dubourdieu, D. (2001). The Color of Odors. *Brain and Language*, 2001.2493.

Movara Fitness Resort. (2015). 7 Types of Eaters - What Type Are You? Retrieved from https://movara.com/7-types-of-eaters-what-type-are-you/

Nourishing. (n.d.). Retrieved from https://www.lifespan.org/lifespan-living/five-myths-intuitive-eating

Peirano, J. (2017). The 6 Different Types of Eaters: Which One Are You? Retrieved from https://www.cheatsheet.com/health-fitness/different-types-of-eaters-which-one-are-you.html/

Please Quit Your Diet, Now. (n.d.). Retrieved from https://www.psychologytoday.com/us/blog/raising-happiness/201203/please-quit-your-diet-now

Psychology of Eating. (n.d.). Retrieved from https://psychologyofeating.com/the-science-and-psychology-of-intuitive-eating/

Psychology of Eating. (n.d.). Retrieved from https://psychologyofeating.com/intuitive-eating/

Rumsey, A. (2019). 24 Intuitive Eating Benefits: Alissa Rumsey Nutrition. Retrieved from https://alissarumsey.com/intuitive-eating/intuitive-eating-benefits/

Spanjers, B. (2018). The Biggest Misunderstandings about Intuitive Eating. Retrieved from https://barbaraspanjers.com/the-biggest-misunderstandings-about-intuitive-eating/

The 10 Principles of Intuitive Eating. (n.d.). Retrieved from http://eatuitive.com/blog/the-10-principles-of-intuitive-eating/

The Five Intuitive Eating Mistakes You're Making. (2019). Retrieved from https://www.ionlycameforthecake.com/five-intuitive-eating-mistakes-youre-making/

Wansink, C. (2005). The office candy dish: proximity's influence on estimated and actual consumption. *International Journal of Obesity*, 871-5.

Made in United States
North Haven, CT
05 November 2026

21769182R10091